First + Shift

Regina M. Callion CEO, MSN, RN

How to Dominate Your First TWO Years of Nursing

TABLE OF CONTENT

1. Introduction   2
2. Dominate the Job Search   4
3. Dominate the Job Interview   15
4. Dominate the Job Interview Look   34
5. Dominate the Job Acceptance Offer   37
6. Dominate the Professional Image   41
   (Nurse uniform basics + Interpersonal relationships)
7. Dominate the Orientation Period   47
8. Dominate the Patient Assignment Report   54
9. Dominate the Patient Introduction   58
10. Dominate the Shift Assignment   61
11. Dominate Speaking (to the Manager, Doctor, and anyone else.)   81
12. Dominate Handoff Report   93
13. Dominate Your Nurse Value   99
14. Dominate Your Nursing Career and Personal life   108
15. Frequently Asked Questions and Answers   123

INTRODUCTION

It is no news that graduating nurses face a lot of challenges that affect successful transition in practice. A lot of healthcare organizations are beginning to come to terms with this reality. However, there's only little they can do. They need to understand how changes in the health care landscape affect new graduate nurses who are transitioning to the next level in their career.

Despite the constant changes in the healthcare system, the need for nurses is on the increase. This demand has become so consistent that more than 20% of immigrants who move to foreign countries are either nurses or others in the medical practice. Clinical practices are faced with increasing pressure to operate in an efficient scope as a result of declining reimbursements, increased consumerism, and a host of other factors. It is now more imperative that education programs produce nurses who will efficiently fit into the work system as soon as they leave school.

As you transition from nursing school to the workforce, you will realize that no matter how prepared you think you are, the challenges in the real world can be quite troublesome. Factors like the increasing number of patients with complex conditions, performance anxiety, overwhelming pressure as a result of the diversity in the workforce, lack of access to experienced mentors and coaches and a host of others are a list of problems that could unsettle new graduate nurses.

As a nurse, we are tasked to care for patients, manage relationships with providers and families, and lead an interprofessional team. If these responsibilities are not accompanied by supportive relationships, new graduate nurses can get overwhelmed and fatigued. Especially if you are a novice, RNs who manage complex patients without adequate support or guide could suffer from anxiety and ultimately lead to quitting nursing.

Healthcare organizations are losing experienced nurses as a result of retirements, pressure from increased workloads, limited resources, and so many others. The new graduate nurse is the key to prevent extinction of the profession. But the issues you will face have to be spoken about frankly and honestly.

Another source of concern for new graduates is workplace bullying. This issue is so debilitating that it obstructs the proper socialization of new nurses. Organizations do little to protect nurses from bullying and by so doing, promote unprofessional behavior. There is a reason why everyone says "Nurses eat their young." Here are ReMar we do the exact opposite! We support, nurture, and care for the young nurse. I was a new nurse not too long ago and I value everything you will bring to the profession.

This self-help book is aimed at mentoring you through your first practice. The first two years of nursing can be tough; that's why you need a guide or a mentor, hence, this book.

DOMINATE YOUR JOB SEARCH

"There is always a part of my mind that is preparing for the worst and another part of my mind that believe if I prepare enough for it, the worst won't happen."

Kay Redfield Jamison

Getting You Equipped as You Start Off Your Nursing Career

It is a common challenge now to run into job openings only to be told it's restricted to those with 5 or more years' experience when you are just a fresh graduate. A lot of human resource firms explain that it's vital to have only experienced medical practitioners working in a hospital. While this can be agreed upon because of the complications that come with the job, it is also vital that you don't get deterred by this standard.

What you do and how much you put into getting your first job will make the big difference in your career. Since you need to keep up with the status quo and dynamics in your field and very importantly, earn enough to pay bills, it is very vital that you engage yourself in the practice. Your dream job should meet you prepared, and by prepared, I mean working in a clinic or hospital. Don't wait around for your dream job take an open position however low profile it seems.

You will be surprised how far your input in that small clinic will go. Since pride doesn't pay bills, don't neglect the "small jobs" as long as you are getting paid for your services. Your dream job is waiting for the experience you gather from the little positions you learn to dominate.

Searching for A Job

There are some keys required to keep you on the right track as you pursue a career in nursing. Most nursing students are lucky if they keep the jobs on their units after a school clinical rotation or internship, but when this does not happen, the following strategies will help when getting a job seems impossible:

❖ **Strategy 1: Self-Assessment**

Before embarking on a job search, first assess your skills and qualifications. Your first battle is knowing who you are and what you can offer. Beside work experiences, there are qualities that separate one person from the other. It may be as simple as how you maintain a relationship with people or the ability to manage a crisis.

List out your clinical and non-clinical skills that are relevant to your search. Then outline your certifications and educational achievements.

These basic lists will equip you in drafting a resume, cover letter, and answer questions during a job interview.

Are you familiar with the SWOT analysis? SWOT stands for Strength, Weaknesses, Opportunities, and Threats. It's a self-help strategy used by some recruiting agencies to discover personal competitive advantages.

Strength and ***Weakness*** are your personal attributes that can either subdue work-related challenges or be buried in them. It is expected that before you read the next chapter, get a note and have this SWOT analysis. List out at least *5 qualities* that you have that you could attribute as a "strength" and do the same about your "weaknesses."

Opportunities describe your abilities as a nurse to adapt to the dynamics in the field of nursing.

Threats are potential negativities or responsibilities that affect your position as a nurse. They include and may not be limited to your proximity to the location of the job, family crisis or divorce, a blemish on your nursing license, illness, and so on.

Another box to check is the condition of the work you are looking for. Find out if it is part time or full time.

❖ **Strategy 2: Job Research**

There used to be times when organizations and human resource (HR) firms would contact potential staffs while they are still in nursing school. Some do it indirectly via the school board. This privilege is only common with Ivy League colleges now and you should not expect to be called for a nursing job.

However, as a fresh graduate or registered nurse, you need to consult the newspapers and online platforms for job openings. Understanding the current job market is a vital part of your search. You need to look out for the organizations hiring, positions that are posted, and the qualifications required for the jobs posted.

Being well informed about job openings is very essential before traveling out of your city, state, or country. There are some online platforms set up with interesting features such as job specification, applicant profile, and the employer's details. LinkedIn is one of the many social platforms that meet these criteria.

Going into the interview with a good understanding of what the organization stands for will give you an advantage. So, endeavor to do advanced research of your own after coming across openings whether in newspapers or online networks. Search for clues about their organizational mission, their vision, accreditation, recognitions received, and achievements. The company's website will be the quickest place to find this information.

Prove to them that you have done your homework as you march into the interview hall with adequate information about your potential employer.

The Job Search Toolbox:

✓ **The Resume**

A very important tool in your toolbox as you begin in searching for opportunities or openings as a nurse is your resume.

A good resume tells the HR or employer all they need to know. This does not mean you have to put down every unnecessary detail that is not relevant to the job.

On most applications that are forwarded online, the resume is commonly requested even though some of its contents have been highlighted in the online application fields.

Whether you submitted your resume online or not, always have a fresh copy of your resume ready to present.

You can also keep various versions of your resume depending on the field you are applying for. Your resume should reflect the position you are applying for. For example, if you are applying to work in pediatrics put on your resume you are seeking a position where you work with children. If you are applying to a cardiac telemetry floor write how you are looking to grow your cardiac experience or exposure to remote telemetry monitoring.

Features of a Resume:

The Heading: this section of your resume should contain the following-

Name and credentials – make it easy to locate your credentials by putting it after your name. You earned it, so don't be shy to flaunt it.

Residential/home address

Email address – remember, every detail is a pointer to who you are. If you have an email that looks like "chainsmokersforreal@yahoo.com," create a new address specifically for your professional career.

Phone Number

Objectives/summary – For your cover letters, applicant objectives should be kept brief and straight to the point. For example, "Skilled registered nurse seeking a position in a neonatal intensive care unit (NICU)." However, on your resume, you can make your summary have more detail. Let it highlight your experience, accomplishments, credentials, and special skills.

Your summary shouldn't be vague or imprecise. It should target the reader that it is intended for.

As a new nurse without clinical experience, you can list out your clinical rotations. When you gain professional experience, your clinical experiences in nursing school will lose value and can be removed from the resume.

Your education should be clearly listed. You can also include non-nursing training if you think it will add value to your presentation.

Sample of Some Resumes

An Entry Level Nursing Assistant: Assistants often face the challenge of drafting a good resume that can compete with other applicant nurses who are more experienced. Having little or no experience shouldn't be a deterrent to drafting a good resume. Even with you little experience, you can parlay related skills into an excellent resume. You can also use some of this terminology to beef up your resume if you worked as a NA.

Alexis Richardson
Brooklyn, NY 13072
(218) 525 2167
Alexis.Richardson@gmail.com

Entry Level Nursing Assistant

Quality Patient Care – Activities of Daily Living – Relationship Building

- Highly motivated to launch nursing career; plan to attend Manhattan Institute's CAN Training Centre in the summer and ultimately pursue RN studies.
- Dedicated, service-focused professional seeking to transition into healthcare as a nursing assistant.
- Backed by a solid work history, reputation as a team player and passion for helping others.
- Background includes experience caring for terminally ill cancer patients.

Professional Experience:

- Primary Care Provider, August, 2013 - September, 2015

Duties:

- Received 'exemplary' and 'exceeds expectations' ratings on all performance reviews. Cited for excellence in interpersonal communications, teamwork, customer service, flexibility and reliability.
- Demonstrated ability to interact with clients from diverse cultures and backgrounds.
- Transformed "difficult" clients into clients who requested me by name.

APPLICATIONS

- Old People's Home (Brooklyn), Volunteer Service
- Humane Society, Volunteer

EDUCATION

- ABC High School, Brooklyn, NY – Graduated with honors

Entry-Level RN: Most top-notch jobs don't just require experience but your certifications as well. Your clinical internships will come in handy when drafting a good resume.

Alexis Richardson, BSN, RN

Miami, Florida 18000 | (515) 801-0155 | Alexis Richardson@livedomain.com | LinkedIn URL

Qualifications Summary

o   Registered Nurse (RN) with specialty experience in psychiatric nursing. Developed strong psychiatric-evaluation and treatment-planning skills through RN role at ABC Department of Corrections. Knowledge of psychotropic medication administration, management and training.

Professional Experience

Registered Nurse, July, 2018 – Present - ABC Department of Corrections, Anytown, PA

Hired as an RN following internship at a hospital within a maximum-security correctional facility housing 3,500 inmates. Assigned to the mental health crisis unit and play a key role on interdisciplinary team of psychiatrists, RNs, social workers and corrections officers.

➢ Helped refine unit policies and procedures in the areas of suicide-watch procedures, safety methods, discharge planning and documentation.

➢ Responded to volatile situations and violent outbreaks, earning the respect of team members for levelheaded and quick thinking to restore the safety and security of patients, staff and inmates.

➢ Completed training in management of assaultive behaviors and psychotropic-medication administration

Student Nurse | Clinical Rotations - DEF Hospital, Anytown, PA

Worked under the supervision of an RN providing bedside care, treatment and clinical documentation for patients on cardiac, oncology and medical-surgical floors.

➢   Treated an average of 16 patients daily double the average student caseload.
➢   Gained experience in procedures such as cryotherapy and trigger-point injections.
➢   Presented in-service training on ethics concerning elderly atrial fibrillation treatment.
➢   Earned a reputation for nursing excellence. Supervisor comments: "Marcy's clinical skills are impressive...she would be an asset to any nursing team."

Nurse Practicum | 150 hours - GHI Hospital, Psychiatric Unit, Anytown, PA

Completed practicum providing nursing care to patients with both acute and chronic mental health issues.

EDUCATION

Bachelor of Science in Nursing (BSN) - ABC College of Nursing, Anytown, PA
Course Highlights: Healthcare Delivery Models, Nursing Health Assessment, Clinical and Chemical Therapeutics, Biophysical Pathology, Psychosocial Pathology, Human Anatomy and Physiology, Statistics, Nursing Research

Registered Nurse, State of Pennsylvania

This a formal letter addressed to your potential employer or human resource team explaining how you received the job opening and your interest to work in a specific position as posted in the opening.

Remember what has been said of a first impression. Since your cover letter is always the first item in view, it is important to avoid mistakes or unnecessary details that may kill the interest to read the entire application.

It should always be printed on the same paper, with a uniformed font and general style as your resume.

It should also have the same heading contact information at the top of the page.

On the recipient's block, address the specific person to whom your letter is addressed. In most cases, getting the recipient's name can be very tricky. If that is the case, get the title of the recipient who will be reviewing your resume. If the recipient is more than one individual or their title remains difficult to find out, you can address them as "Human Resource Manager" or "Nurse Manager."

✓ Body of The Letter

Start off the first paragraph by stating your purpose of writing and the position you are applying for. Express your desire or specific interest for that position while you carefully take a positive hint about their organization.

The following paragraphs should be as precise as possible. Tell them about your skills, education, knowledge, or experience that separates you from any other candidate for the position.

You can use the cover letter to explain some abridged information you listed in your resume. Where your resume fails to highlight, your cover letter *covers* it for you.

Your closing paragraph should reiterate your enthusiasm and interest. Thank the recipient or organization for their interest.

✓ Closing/Salutation

End the letter with a professional salutation. A good example is "Sincerely yours" etc.

21, August, 2019

Charisse Palmer RN
153 Main Street
Manhattan, New York City

Cara Lee, RN, C, MSN
Nurse Recruiter
NYU Langone Medical Center
Manhattan, New York

Dear Ms. Lee:

I am responding to your advertisement for staff that appeared in the July, 2019 issue of Nursing Spectrum. As listed in my attached resume, I have a strong background in clinical specialty area(s) nursing.

I have molded my career from its inception to achieve my goal of becoming a Registered Nurse. My experience and education have provided me with excellent knowledge of patient assessment and treatment including medical surgical practices, acute patient care and patient relations. This, coupled with my attention to detail, organizational and communication skills will allow me to make a substantial contribution to NYU Langone Medical Centre.

I believe that a challenging environment such as yours will provide an excellent opportunity for me to best utilize my skills while contributing to the healthcare community, patients and their families.

I welcome the opportunity to discuss with you personally how my skills and strengths can best serve your hospital. I will call you the week of September 2019 to establish a convenient time for us to meet and further discuss my qualifications. I look forward to learning more about NYU Langone Medical Center and the possibility of becoming a part of your team.

Sincerely,

Charisse Palmer, RN.

MARQUIS CLIFF, RN

25 Main Street
New Cityland, CA 37610
Cell: (555) 319-7893
Email: cliff_marquis@live.com

Dear Hiring Manager,

I am interested in the Registered Nurse position available St. Luke Roosevelt Hospital Centre. As a Registered Nurse licensed to practice in California and with 5 months experience, I believe that I am well suited for this position.

In the course of caring for female patients of all ages, I have become proficient in assessing vitals, collecting specimens and administering medications. I have also had the chance to:

- Educate patients on post-operative medications and total wellness care.
- Help pregnant patients optimize health through diet and exercise choices.
- Assist doctors with in-office surgeries and non-invasive procedures.
- Train new staff on office quality and regulatory procedures.

Additionally, I have expertise in HIPPA rules and have been in charge of office procedural updates to ensure total regulatory compliance.

You will find my resume and a list of references attached. Please feel free to contact me at your earliest convenience so we can discuss the position and your needs in detail.

Sincerely,

Marquis Cliff

A business card is a miniature customized resume that you can carry with you anywhere. It is designed to contain your name and other vital information about you and your services.

Sometimes, you can run into an old-time friend, former business partner, or a well- connected professional in a social or formal setting. At such times, it is expedient to give them your business card. Apart from the potential benefit that comes with giving out business cards, it also demonstrates that you're a savvy professional in your field.

Your business card should be two-sided; the front page containing your name, credentials, and contact information. Behind it, you can list your skill sets and qualities that distinguish you as a nurse.

✓ **Digital Platforms**

Another essential tool is your digital presence. A potential employer can get information about you on the internet.

The advantages that social media handles like Facebook, Instagram, or Twitter handle presents are enormous. Via these platforms, you could connect with a potential employer faster and easier.

As a matter of fact, some employers take their time to research on their potential staffs before or after an interview. This will present them access to your profile and identification. Therefore, it is also vital that you create a spotless online content. Be careful about what you post. Even after deleting a picture, it is possible that a user might have saved the item for reference. Besides, there's nothing you post online that is actually ever deleted. Smart hackers can use powerful software to retrieve items that were previously deleted.

When I hire for ReMar I always check the applicant's Facebook page for information if I see unprofessional, crude, or inappropriate content it helps to guide my decision if the person will be a good fit for my company.

Human Resource Firms and Recruiting Agencies

This is another platform where employers and job seekers can connect. Staffing agencies and recruiters organize general interviews for various professionals, including nursing. These agencies earn a commission from employers to recruit applicants for positions.

✓ **Job Boards**

As mentioned above in Digital Platforms, there are several online platforms that are created for the sole purpose of connecting job seekers with employers.

They start out by posting general services providing for all job seekers until they started catering to very specific specialties. Hospitals and healthcare employers have their own job boards.

However, a lot of these job boards duplicate their posts. For instance, a hospital could post a nursing job on their website and also duplicate the same to HealthCareers.com. Other job board sites could pick up the same job category making multiple duplications of the job.

As a result, latest job sites like Indeed.com integrate these networks with job boards. So, to avoid missing out on opportunities, you can subscribe to hospital websites and reliable sites like. This will make it easy for you to access new jobs immediately when they are posted.

Most of these sites allow users to upload their resumes. It's vital that you register and upload your resume on each one you subscribe to.

Other important things to do as you register for these job sites:

Create an email address for job search. This makes sense because of the tons of spam messages that clog your regular email address. Filling in your email address to these job boards makes it vulnerable for spam messages. So, it's wise to separate your primary email address from the one you have created for the job sites. You wouldn't want to search through your regular email address with tons of messages looking for fresh updates from the job sites you registered with.

Sign up for job alerts with the reliable aggregators and hospital sites you have registered with. Keep in mind that not all sites have job alert systems.

DOMINATE THE JOB INTERVIEW

"The man who has confidence in himself gains the confidence of others."

Hasidic Proverb

Gateways to Securing the Job

Unlike most interviews organized for corporate office jobs, interviews for nursing jobs are different. It takes a lot of preparation and practice to secure a nursing job. But that shouldn't discourage you because you've done the hardest part by getting through nursing school.

The fact that you made it to an interview means that your paperwork was very satisfactory. Your potential employer just wants to be convinced that all you put in your resume is true, and you can help them reach their goals.

It is also an opportunity to assess your role and potential employer. Does the working condition suit your profile and core values? Can it help you reach your goal? Your evaluation should inform you if the job is actually enjoyable. That is what this process is about remember your life is determined by your decisions. You should always remain in control of what you will do.

Employers have their various interviewing strategies and processes. Some are conducted via a telephone conversation, video calls, or directly at job fairs. These kinds of interviews are short and usually conducted by the hiring manager.

The objective is to reduce the number of candidates and invite the best candidates for the next step in the process.

These interviewers are either recruiters or a team of staffs from the Human Resource Department. They are very skilled at asking short, straightforward questions to quickly obtain the details they need.

Ensure you give the right answers that will convince them to send you to the next stage.

First + Shift

Remember you are qualified for the job. The goal here is to know you in person and to see if you are as good as you look on paper. Another thing they look out for (although not mandatory) is to find out if your personality suits the rest of the team.

The following are tips on how to prepare for In-Person Interviews:

1) Take Notes

During your self-assessment, as explained in the first chapter, it is recommended that you write down those facts during the exercise. It is common to resort to electronic gadgets, but studies have shown that putting down note with pen and paper leaves a lasting impression in the memory.

So, while you do your SWOT analysis, carefully list out those weaknesses, strength, opportunities, and threats that you can find.

2) Assess and Compare

When you come across the job posting, the first thing you should do is to assess and compare them with your credentials. It is not a time to skim through the passage. You have to read it thoroughly to avoid skipping essential details.

You can analyze them carefully by listing the qualifications the employer is seeking on one side. Then, list your skills, credentials, and accomplishments that meet the employer's needs on the other side. This analytical style will help you remember these details and boost your confidence during the interview.

It's also imperative that you know your goals and what you can contribute to the organization.

3) Find Out More About the Job

Don't settle for the job posting and assessment alone. The more you know about the job and the organization, the better.

All you need to know about the organization and its facilities is available on their website. Your interviewers expect you to do your homework in this aspect and will dish out questions to test your knowledge. For example, when I hire for ReMar the first question I like to ask is what do you know about us?

16

Research their facilities, accomplishments, what they represent, their mission, goals, and objectives.

Most candidates go into an interview entirely in the dark about the company, and as a result, they lose confidence during the interview process. Your interviewer will know if you've researched them because they will ask specific questions about their hospital.

4) Check Their Social Handles

Organizations, including hospitals, have some form of social base. The proliferation of social media has made a lot of these organizations accessible online.

Beside looking them up on their website, you should also check them on Facebook, Instagram, Twitter, or LinkedIn to know their values and culture.

5) Read Reviews and Feedbacks from other Nurses

Some websites make provision for feedbacks and professional reviews. Although this is not very common with hospitals because of the confidential stakes involved.

However, there are platforms where patients and employees of a hospital could leave reviews about their hospital facilities, condition, environment and personal experiences. You can look out for online nursing forums to see what your colleagues are saying.

6) Research Specifics such as Salary and Schedules

It's unusual for employees to reveal their salaries on social media platforms or online forums. But you can play the detective by digging deep into their conversations or consulting members directly on their page.

Find out about their work schedules and working conditions.

7) Have a Safe Social Media Profile

Social media is a boundless world where people connect for both social and corporate reasons. The same way you can access your potential employer via social media also applies to you.

Again, your social media accounts could be the first place your potential employer will look at before considering you for a job. You have to clean up your account and ensure it is free of any negativity that might ruin your chances of securing the job. Let your social media profile(s) be the best reflection of you even before you submit your resume.

8) Avoid Clichés

You have prepared for the job. You have all your documents ready, you've done your research, but the only thing in the way of securing your job is an intelligent expression.

Remember, the difference between you and the interviewers is time. Don't lose your esteem to anxiety. Someday, it could be you sitting on their chair, asking the questions. Compose yourself and be original. Don't subscribe to stereotypical way of thinking. People will choose original over phonies any day.

You will definitely come across a zillion articles suggesting ways to pass an interview. While it is okay to read them, it's not wise to rehearse the answers they suggest. This book is in your hand to mentor you into accomplishing your dreams as a nurse without being subdued by the everyday challenges encountered by your senior nursing colleagues in their first year.

In this chapter, some common questions and smart answers will be provided. However, try to assure your employer that you can resolve problems in many ways regardless of the case. It's your job to make them believe in your ideas.

9) Dress the part

Before you open your lips, before that lovely smile, the first thing in view is how you dress. Dressing smartly and neatly is a fundamental attribute in the nursing career.

Your body language also plays a significant role in creating a lasting impression. As a result, you need to watch yourself answering questions in a mirror.

You can also ask your friends who are more experienced to act as interviewers. They should be honest in their judgment of you. Your interviewers are interested in your posture, facial expressions, and other non-verbal cues.

While you sit for your interview, sit up straight with both feet on the floor. Keep your eyes forward, and shoulders squared towards your audience.

Your interviewers are likely to ask you behavioral questions to examine your non-verbal cues. This is a frequent tactic healthcare employer use in their interviews.

Answering Interview Questions

To detect your behavior, your interviewers will ask you behavioral questions. Be smart enough to give honest answers that are devoid of stereotype. An intelligent way of doing this is the use of storytelling. It's a powerful strategy that also invokes memory.

Make sure your story provides evidence that supports your statements in your cover letter and resume.

Storytelling gives you an escape route when you are stuck by a question. It also gives life to your statements as contained in your resume.

However, there are rules in storytelling to avoid spinning into fictions or just plain lying.

You should ensure you remain concise and specific about the steps you took and the lessons you learned from the circumstance.

There's a communication process known as the STAR technique, an acronym representing the four components of communication in nursing.

Situation – WHAT WAS THE EXACT SITUATION? WHO WERE INVOLVED? WHY DID THE SITUATION HAPPEN?

Task or **Target** – WHY WERE YOU INVOLVED IN THE TASK? WHAT IS THE BACKGROUND STORY?

Action – WHAT STEPS DID YOU TAKE TO RESOLVE THE SITUATION? WHY DID YOU CHOOSE TO COMPLETE THE TASK?

Result – WHAT WAS THE OUTCOME? HOW DID YOU FEEL ABOUT THE RESULT? WHAT ARE YOUR LESSONS? HOW DID THE SITUATIONS INFLUENCE WHO YOU AE TODAY?

It is designed to enable you to provide a meaningful and complete answer to questions. Many interviewers have been trained to use the STAR technique.

First Step - Situation or Task

Here you are asked to describe the situation you were confronted with or the task that needed to be completed. Using the STAR technique, you need to set the context. Make it informative and concise, focusing on what is useful to the story. For instance, if the question is asking you to describe where you had to deal with a difficult person, explain how you met the person and why they were difficult. If the question has to do with teamwork, explain the task that you had to undertake as a team.

To begin your story, describe the situation you faced by painting a specific picture of the situation.

Sample: It was the first day of my routine nursing assignment. I met my first patient, Denise, and she was doing well coping with her labor. I was happy awaiting the birth of her daughter, April. Her boyfriend, Dre, was very matured in the way he managed the situation."

BACKGROUND (TASK)

Explain your specific role in the task. Remember you are giving the background story.

"After about 15 minutes of monitoring the baby's heartbeat, I noticed that it was dropping."

Second Step - ACTION

This is the most essential step of the STAR technique because it is where you will need to explain and highlight the skills and personal attributes that the question is testing.

Since you have set the context of your story, you need to explain WHAT you did. To get this done, you need to have these in mind:

Be personal in your approach; talk about you, not the entire team.

Be detailed in your explanation. Don't assume that they can guess what you mean.

Avoid the technicalities involved in the situation unless it is very necessary.

Demonstrate what your actions, how you did it, and your reasons.

Also, have it in mind that your interviewers want to know how you reacted to the situation. It is not a movie script, just be natural.

Sample: "To avoid causing panic, I assured Denise that her baby was okay. I explained to her that her baby may not enjoy laying on the right side, so I guided her onto her left side and requested that she take slow, deep breaths. After observing the situation for a few minutes, there was no increase, so I turned Denise back to the right side. Her baby's heartbeat did not increase. I asked Dre to coach her breathing to calm her nerves.

This was when I involved the midwife and continued to coach Denise through her breathing. Her midwife, Melissa, decreased the Pitocin and explained to Denise that if the baby's heart rate does not remain normal she would be sent for an emergency cesarean section."

Third Step – Result

Here you explain what eventually happened. Tell the audience how it ended and also use the opportunity to describe what you accomplished.

Highlight your lessons from the entire experience. This will help answer the question of personal skills.

Keep in mind that your creativity or expertise is observed at this stage. The interviewers want to know how you were able to resolve the situation using a variety of generic skills in to achieve your objectives.

State the outcome of your actions in detail and highlight your strengths.

Sample: "My keen observation and care helped in the vaginal birth of a gorgeous baby girl named April. I have remained in contact with Denise and her family on WhatsApp. She often sends me the photos of April, who is now 2 years old.

"Eventually, I extended my contract at the facility and became a Charge Nurse. I learned that building a strong connection with a patient from the onset can have positive lasting results. That's just who I am."

Note that, the interviewers are not necessarily interested in your heroic efforts. They don't expect you to be performing emergency cardiac surgery with a drinking straw or some other movie like rescue. They are listening to learn more about you and your skills. They want to know more about your responsibilities, self-awareness, thought process, and past experiences. Like NCLEX, they want to know if you are a <u>safe nurse</u>.

<u>Common Nursing Interview Questions</u>

Most interviewees flunk at interviews because they cram some answers to some of these questions without giving it examples from their personal experience.

The nursing profession is not the regular entrepreneurship outfit that requires a general approach. You can't have answers ready for common questions. Good answers are specific and draw from our personal experience or real-life instances.

To answer most of the questions for nursing interviews rightly, ensure you have:

(i)   Read the job descriptions and all its requirements,

(ii)   Evaluated your accomplishments that prove you are suitable for the job

(iii)   Practiced with self exercises (in the form of rehearsals) that will test your ability to answer nursing interview questions.

Here are some typical nursing interview questions you will probably come across.

1) **Amongst all other lucrative professions, why did you choose to be a nurse?**

This is one of the most common questions asked by recruiters and interviewers. Of course, nursing is a demanding profession. Nurses deal with life-threatening risks almost on a daily basis. They face fear, hardship, and frustration, virtually on a regular basis. But people still troop into the profession nonetheless. Our reasons might be different, but it takes a good reason to determine if one can last long in this profession despite the challenges that come with it.

Don't try too hard to give a smart answer. Your genuine reasons are adequate enough.

Smart Answer:

I take joy in caring for others. It's a trait I discovered early in my life. Nursing is my passion. I always had a pet growing up and that is really how I know I discovered nursing early. Caring for my pets was a natural training ground.

As I grew older, I discovered that I wanted to do something challenging, exciting, and makes a difference in the life of people.

In the nursing profession, we deal with many aspects of patient care. I also enjoy the variety in the routine.

Tip: This is a smart answer because the interviewer will be impressed, having found out that the candidate strives to make a difference in people's lives. And the interviewer may also be able to relate if they had pets as well growing up. 2 points for you!

2) **Tell me About Yourself**

Another popular question at most interviews. The interviewer wants to know details of your person. As easy as it may sound, the administrator wants to know your personality traits as it relates to your nursing career.

The hidden question in the statement is actually, "why are you perfect for this job?" Don't make the mistake of taking a generic approach to this question. Your answer should reflect some of your skills, accomplishments, and what distinguishes you from other candidates for the job.

Smart Answer:

I'm just finishing up nursing school. I've got a 3.85 GPA, and I received an award for the Most Outstanding Undergraduate Nursing Student.

During my internship at Metropolitan Hospital Center, I received frequent commendations from the supervisor for my efficiency. For patient education, I also maintained 93% positive evaluations.

I've also worked as a CNA for a year at Metropolitan Hospital Center. My manager there wants to retain me because of my strong work ethic and my interpersonal skills. I would love to work for her, but I'm excited about being a nurse here at Lenox Hill Hospital. Your commitment to patient education and ongoing staff training is perfect for my skills and drive.

Tip: Make sure you put up an impressive answer from the stat. Your chance of getting hired depends on your preparation and rehearsals.

3) **Have you ever handled a difficult patient? How was your experience?**

This is another likely question to come up. It is a common experience for nurses to come across difficult patients. The difficult patient can have a range of issues. It could be they are refusing to take their medication or they just have a very busy treatment schedule which makes time management stressful.

Look for the most interesting experience you've had in your past and narrate it using the STAR technique.

Smart Answer:

If someone is difficult, there's always a reason for it. Respectfully treating people can often have surprising outcomes.

I once had a client who got a reputation on the unit for being quite rude to the nurses who were responsible for his care. In handoff report I learned Mr. Brown was a retired veteran who lost both legs in a war. When I first met him, I wasn't aware that he liked his water room temperature so when I brought in a cup of ice. I thought I was being a wonderful nurse by doing so I was shocked at his response. He told me that if he had legs he would kick me in the behind for bringing that ice in his room.

Perhaps the other nurses got offended by comments like that but I was not. I asked Mr. Brown what about the ice upset him? I told him I liked room temperature water too but I was interested to know about his preference.

Mr. Brown told me that when he lost his legs they used ice as a therapy and now he couldn't stand the sight of ice due to post traumatic stress. That information gave me an opportunity to have a meaningful conversation with my patient.

I then told him about how my grandfather lost his leg in the war but still continued to live a full life as a Pastor of two churches. From then on Mr. Brown and I had a positive nurse-patient relationship.

4) **What are your strengths and weaknesses?**

You've already had a personal SWOT exercise, so this question shouldn't pose a problem for you. However, amongst your several strength and weaknesses, concentrate on the ones that suit the job profile.

Use your real-life experiences or instances that prove them.

For example, if the job values compassion and problem solving above all other skills, below is an excellent example of how to answer the question of strengths and weaknesses.

Smart Answer:

My biggest strength is compassion and the ability to solve difficult problems. I can narrate so many instances, but one of the interesting cases was about a teenage boy who had terrible nightmares. As a result, he would often wake up after a short nap calling for his mom. This persisted for a while, and it became worrisome for other patients that needed a bit of peace and quiet, especially at nights.

His mom worked two jobs and therefore, could not be in the hospital most of the time. So, she had her younger sister, Eva come to look after him. Unfortunately, the problem was too much, even for his aunt.

I learned about his case during my night shifts. I took an interest in learning what his nightmares were about. I was able to deduce where the problem originated. He was often abused by his stepfather and had to keep it bottled up to preserve his mother's marriage.

His need for hospital treatment was a result of the abuse, but he told his mom it was an accident. I was able to connect with him because I am very familiar with child abuse and the devastating effect it could have on kids.

I a lot of my working hours with him. He felt comfortable telling me everything he couldn't tell his mom. I told him that I had to report this issue for his safety and that he had not done any wrong. I told him he was smart and brave for asking for help. I told him his medical condition would help to secure a proper investigation would take place. His nightmares became less frequent. I can also report that his mother was receptive to the hospital counselor and took appropriate action to protect her son.

My biggest weakness is that I get irritated with colleagues who are too relaxed about issues that require urgent actions. In many cases nurses can become desensitized to medical needs because of our constant exposure. But to that one patient the matter of immediate action or response could be life or death. For example, if I client is stating they have a headache some nurses will say "It is just a call for Tylenol." However, the client could be experiencing a hypertensive crisis and not know it.

Tip: The strength as narrated in the story depicts a compassionate nurse who is willing to go the extra mile in solving a problem. It suits the job profile. The weakness is also understandable as it shows work ethic.

5) Where Do You See Yourself in 5 years?

Beneath this question is the real question of whether you love the job enough to stick with it.

You should make it clear that it's your dream job. Tell them how much you want to learn from the superior staffs in the hospital and your ambition to climb the ladder.

Note that, giving a credible answer to this question depends on how well you know the job. So, do your research on the job specification and the hospital facilities.

Smart Answer:

In five years, I would like to be a reference point as far as the nursing profession is concerned. I want to be the most valued nurse on your team.

I have a burning desire to improve my skills in patient education and electronic health records, and since Lenox Hill Hospital offers education reimbursement, I intend on taking advantage of it.

There are so many new skills I'd like to acquire, and this hospital is a perfect place to nurture and develop myself into a better nurse.

6) Why are You the Best Person for this Nursing Job?

This question also requires a good knowledge of what the job is about. You may also need to talk to other nurses who work there. Find out the challenges they face.

Smart Answer:

I know your major concern presently is efficient budgeting. With my experience at San Juan Medical, Puerto Rico I believe I can resolve these challenges. When I was at Presbyterian Hospital, I was placed in a team tasked to fix our budgeting problems. We were able to reduce inventory costs by 16.3% while ensuring an increase in budget satisfaction.

My team and I were able to:

- Track down inventory and thereby improving productivity.
- Review contacts for equipment and service providers. This helped to save cost.
- We made sure the finance department were in the loop as we explained every budgetary decision we made.
- reduce readmission rates by making sure patients attend post-acute office visits after being discharged.
- improve deficiencies in the emergency room.
- maintain a warranty database.

7) What Do You Find Most Rewarding About Nursing?

The objective of this question is to test your passion. If you see great rewards in the profession, you will also be perceived to be powerful as well.

Smart Answer:

The reward for nursing is boundless. The feeling of seeing your patients improve makes you sleep well at night. It is bigger than monthly paycheck.

Can you imagine getting paid for what you enjoy doing? It's like being paid for loving your kids. Helping people feel better is the best thing I've ever done. I can't tell what could be more rewarding than being the reason for someone's health improvement.

Tip: You can also use a story to make your point. Demonstrate how nursing ties into your everyday life.

8) **What is your Strongest Skill as a Nurse?**

Your background knowledge will come in handy for nurse interview questions like this. The administrators are testing you to know if you will fit into their team. Assuming their most significant need is better patient education, and that's your strongest skill, you're hired.

You should mention at least three, starting with your strongest skills.

Smart Answer:

I thrive well with patient education, stress management, and interpersonal skills. My strongest is in patient education. Being able to calm the fears of my patients is one of my strongest suits.

On one occasion, a patient was unable to reduce his blood pressure following a heart attack. I was charged with the responsibility to educate him about diet and exercise. I did research about patients with a similar condition who had changed their routines.

The outcome was successful that he even sent me postcards 4 months after his discharge.

Tip: Be honest in your answers. If you don't have experience or a particular skill just say so. Tell the interviewer that you are excited to learn. Honesty might be the only key that lands you the job. No one is a fan of falsehood.

9) **How Do You Deal with the Stress of Nursing?**

Stress is a common feature in the nursing profession. Administrators want to know you've got the strength to push through tough times especially if you could possibly be eaten alive by the senior staff. The question is meant to test your ability to handle stress on all fronts. It is not abnormal to vent frustrations at times if it is done in a healthy and HIPAA-compliant ways.

Smart Answer:

As sweet as the nursing profession is, dealing with stress is also part of the job. During my days as a nursing student, we lost a 14-year-old boy to cancer on one of my clinical units. It was one of the most traumatic experience I've had in my career to date. Bonding with my patients is something I can't help. It had an effect on me emotionally until I decided to join a support group.

Speaking about it and imbibing the strategies for dealing with stress that I learned from the group helped me immensely. An emotional support group is my go-to for managing stress.

10) What's the Hardest Thing About Being A Nurse?

A Nursing job is not easy. Questions like this are intended to test your honesty and ability to handle the job. You will upset them if you say it isn't hard. However, when you admit that it is hard, cite examples of common challenges in the nursing profession and then offer your solutions it will make a lasting impact.

Smart Answer

The tricky part of the job is the physicality involvement. Standing on my feet for an entire 12-hours shift can take a toll on my body. Sometimes I have to deny myself breaks just to stay on top of the responsibilities. This is the tough side of nursing that school didn't prepare me for. However, I always get back on my feet after a good rest and regular exercises.

I've also joined a Zumba class, and it's been very helpful because of the stress-relieving exercises involved.

The above 10 questions are the most common interview questions you will likely come across.

Below are additional 20 questions to prep you up to dominate your interview. Get a note and a pen and list out your smart answers for each of them.

11) Why did you leave your last job?

12) Why should we hire you?

13) Are you at ease working with other nurses and doctors?

14) Why do you want to work here?

15) How did you hear about the job?

16) What is your proudest accomplishment as a nurse, and why?

17) Would you call yourself a team player?

18) Tell us about a time you worked with a difficult colleague. How did you handle the situation? Were you able to build a relationship with the person?

19) Have you handled a leadership role? How did you manage?

20) Have you ever caused conflict (accidentally)? What happened, and how did you handle it?

21) Have you ever had to do something exceptional that makes you proud?

22) Have you had experience with a very ill patient that required your time? How did you manage to attend to the patient while also ensuring your other patients were adequately cared for?

23) Tell us about a time you identified upcoming problems with a patient?

24) Was there ever a time you didn't know how to handle a healthcare issue? How was it resolved?

25) Tell us about a time you effectively educated a patient or their relative on difficult medical jargon.

26) Was there ever a time you had to persuade a patient about something? Tell us how.

27) Was there ever a time when a patient's family was dissatisfied with your care? How did you handle the situation?

28) Tell us about a time you worked in a fast-paced setting. How did you prioritize tasks while maintaining excellent patient care?

29) Tell us about a challenging situation or problem where you took an exemplary role to correct it instead of waiting for someone else to fix it.

30) How do you balance your work and your personal life?

Questions You Should Ask in a Nursing Interview

Your interviewers are likely to ask you if you have any questions. Answer in the affirmative. This is another opportunity to show you are engaged in the process. To have zero questions for the prospective employers mean you don't have any insight to gain from your own investigative position. In other words, it looks bad!

Asking the administrators questions about the organization or the job gives you a chance to learn about the opening.

The following are some questions you can ask your interviewer:

1)   **What kind of training do you offer?** Most reputable hospitals offer a variety of training for nurses. By asking this question, it convinces your administrators of your intention to stick around for a long time.

2)   **What's your policy for tuition reimbursement**? Just like the first question, this also shows your interest and determination to stay long in the job.

3)   **What do other nurses like most about working here?** This is another vital question that you should ask to find out interesting facts about the hospital. You might have missed the chance to know them during your research on the job.

4)   **What's the culture like here?** Every organization has ways of doing things. Finding out the true facts may demand that you ask someone on the inside.

It also shows your interest and enthusiasm to learn and understand the job.

5) How do you measure nursing success? The definition of success varies according to individuals. Some define success by material achievement, while others describe it as the number of people your life has impacted.

And of course, asking an important question like this goes to show the kind of person you are.

Other questions you can ask

6) **How about your staffing ratios?**
7) **What kind of system do you use for EMR?**
8) **What's your requirement for weekend rotation?**
9) **How long are the shifts?**
10) **What's your policy on overtime?**

Asking these questions shows you've thought through the most challenging aspect of the job.

Essential Interview Tips

✓ Be sincere when answering interview questions. Your interviewers are experts and have probably been participating in the recruiting process for a long time. They could ask you follow-up questions to ascertain if your answers are true. If they suspect you're lying, you have jeopardized your chances of getting hired.

✓ You should dress professionally. It takes more than smart answers to land the job. You must look the part too. (This will be discussed further in the third chapter).

✓ Make adequate preparation before your interview. Rehearse your nursing interview questions. Don't skim through.

✓ Get enough rest. Also, eat and hydrate well too.

✓ Know where you're going to avoid looking for confused when you get there. This is because some healthcare facilities can be quite big and confusing.

Knowing the exact location will also help you to get good rest the night before by reducing an aspect to cause anxiety.

Items to come along with to your interview

The following are items to bring on your interview;

- A. Copies of your resume
- B. Copies of nursing license and other certifications
- C. Letter of reference
- D. Your business card(s)
- E. Folders to contain a copy of each item listed above to be handed to each interviewer.
- F. A pen and notepad

FOLLOW UP

This stage is not necessary, but it speaks volume of who you are. Besides, a good follow up has the potential of overturning an average interview.

Send a thank you card. Stand out from the others by sending one. If you feel it's too much, you can send a simple email.

IF you do not get feedback from the Human Resource team after the time they gave you has elapsed and you are still interested in the job, follow them up via email or call their line.

DOMINATE THE JOB INTERVIEW LOOK

"The way to gain a good reputation is to endeavor to be what you desire to appear."

Socrates

Creating a Physical Impression

There are a few places where opinions matter and one of them is at your interview. Opinions are often the products of what we see, hear, or perceive. Opinions will be formed whether we permit it or not.

The quintessential image of the nursing profession encompasses their dress culture, work ethic, and professionalism.

When you are trying to figure out what to wear for a nursing interview, it's normal to be confused. This may be a result of nervousness or the conflicting messages that emanates from the preparation for the interview. You might be stuck with the choice to either look simple, casual or try to impress your audience.

Does it matter what you wear to a nursing interview then? Absolutely!

Your appearance might be the deciding factor between whether you land the job or not. First impressions should never be taken for granted, especially if it has to do with interviews for a job. It is natural for people to go with the visual cues – your look, posture, expression, etc.

In a social setting, appearance says a lot about who we are. People put in a lot of efforts trying to impress a new person in their life on a date. This is because opinions will be formed at the initial state and consequently will be used as a viewpoint to create a conclusion on the individual.

People can relate more with nurses more than other fields in the field of medicine.

Decency, neatness, and humility are somewhat like a culture with nurses. So, if you are going to a nursing interview for the job, you better dress the part.

As generic as it may sound, your interviewer may also have the same perception. It is in human nature to judge from what we see.

A common myth you should discard is the notion that you might be interviewed by a nurse, so they will understand if you dress casually. Unfortunately, that's often not the case. There's a big chance that the interview will be conducted by either member of the human resource, nurse administrator, or experienced recruiters who are not nurses.

Attires That Shouldn't Make It to the Interview

1) Revealing clothes. It's totally unprofessional. Perhaps you should save it for your social settings.
2) High heeled shoes. These are also not professional for the situation. Nurses are safety conscious, and wearing high heeled shoes do not demonstrate safety.
3) Poorly fitting clothes. If it's too tight or too loose, change it.
4) Tennis shoes or sneakers. Save for it for your casual settings.
5) Untidy ironed/pressed clothes. This betrays the neatness culture in nursing.
6) Excessive makeup, cologne, or perfume. Be moderate with those.
7) Unkempt hair or not being groomed. Bath and comb your hair.

Attires that can make it to the interview

While it is important to make an impression in your interview, you should also be moderate. Don't go over the top trying to impress the administrators.

Your objectives are to make a good impression and more importantly, get the job.

Here are some suggestions of what to wear to your interview:

- Professional business attire.

Clothes:

FOR MEN

- Fitted jackets or blazer.
- Necktie.
- Slacks.

FOR WOMEN

- A blouse.
- A skirt.
- A button-down sweater
- Slacks would also be appropriate.

Shoes:

MEN

- Dark-colored dress shoes or shoes that match your dress.

WOMEN

- Polished and clean pumps or flats.

Accessories and jewelry

Keep it simple.

Remember: Under no circumstances should you wear <u>scrubs</u> to a job interview. They are not appropriate for the interview even if you will spend most of your life in them after you get the job.

DOMINATE THE JOB ACCEPTANCE OFFER

"The tragedy of life is not found in failure but complacency. Not in you doing too much, but doing too little. Not in your living above your means, but below your capacity. It's not failure but aiming too low, that is life's greatest tragedy."

Benjamin E. Mays

Post-Interview Processes

Don't ever entertain the idea of getting complacent at this stage. A good interview does not present a 100% guarantee that the job is secured. This is why you should endeavor to follow-up on your administrators after an interview.

When the question is not "when can you start?" they will probably assure you of a call-back or a promise to get back to you after the interview.

On securing the job, there are some processes you should still engage to ensure you've maximized the opportunity.

During the offer process, there are a few standard steps to expect. Some of which are verbal notification of job offer in a short while after your interview. Unless you've been given a timeline for the notice, there's no reason for them to delay the process. However, your follow-up on the matter will not just act as a reminder, but will also register your unrelenting desire to work with the organization.

The next step they are likely to take is to notify you via a phone call or email, followed by a formal call to receive your job offer. You should receive a letter from the administrators formally congratulating you and highlighting your official offer.

It is your responsibility to review the offer to make sure if it's right for you. If it doesn't meet your satisfaction, you can renegotiate for a better offer.

Below are various phases or steps during your job offer process.

1) **First phase: The Informal Notification**

Not long after the interview, you will get an informal notification from the unit responsible for the employment process. This notification is to keep you expectant of the offer. This notification is often communicated in the form of a proposition, that is, they will urge you to tell them what exactly you need from them to accept an offer.

If this is not the case, they might send you an email indicating what they are offering you. Notifications like this vary depending on the impression you've made on them. Your response to their notification should begin with appreciation. Then proceed to discuss important items such as pay, bonuses, benefits, working hours, and other important details you need to know.

2) **Second Phase: Official Offer Review**

After the first phase, you are expected to get an official offer letter from the employer. Ensure that the offer comes in written form. If it initially came in the form of a phone call, demand a written document for you to review.

Having it in written form makes it official and easily accessible for reference purpose. Contained in the letter should be your role, start date, benefits, and other vital information to get you started.

By reviewing the content of the letter, you should be able to understand your role as a nurse in your new organization.

Also, if you come across details that are confusing or unacceptable to you, you can call their attention or negotiate with the employer. Remember once you agree to the job you have to work it, so make sure it is really what you want.

3) **Phase Three: Responding to the Job Offer**

Begin by expressing your appreciation. It could go this way – "Thank you for the offer. I'm looking forward to reviewing the terms. When do you need my feedback?" They will need your response to the offer, and if they ask you to respond immediately, you should politely ask for a day to go over the terms.

It is common for new graduate nurses to get too excited at this stage and rush up the process. That may not be ideal because of instances of some certain terms and condition that has been unfair to nurses. Getting this sorted out during this stage should take precedence over any form of celebration arrangements.

Furthermore, proofread your response severally to spot any errors. You can get a friend or a mentor to assist you with this. Prepare and rehearse your response and be ready for any questions or further negotiations.

Here's a letter sample of a job acceptance (that you could send via postage or an email) –

August 18, 2021

Mr. Raymond Lecter
Manager Human Resource
ABC Clinic
106 Main Street
New Cityland, CA 83410

Dear Lecter,
I appreciate your call and for considering my request for a written offer. Thank you for the position of a Practical Nurse. I'm writing to formally accept your conditions of employment that you mentioned in the offer letter.

Per our discussion, my full-time starting salary will be $65,400 per year with a three-week paid vacation. I am aware that my health plans will begin upon start date with the option of a flexible spending account.

Today, I tendered my immediate resignation at Louisville Hospital. Therefore, I will be able to resume work on September 2nd, 2021.

I am honored that your organization considers me experienced to work in your ICU operations, and I will work diligently to deliver the results we discussed. I am eager to handle all duties at ABC Clinic, including medication administration, patient education, emotional and physical support, and assuring that the overall quality of care adheres to the hospital's standard.

I look forward to receiving my job contract and a copy of my job description, which I will sign and return promptly. I anticipate that our work relationship will be positive and long-lasting; I see myself working well with your clinic and its staff, and I am excited about my first day at work. If there is any further information that you need from me, please feel free to ask.

Thank you for your confidence and support.

Sincerely,

Donna Hughes

Negotiating A Job Offer

A significant aspect of the acceptance process is negotiating the items in the job offer, its terms, and conditions. Also, use the opportunity to negotiate your salary and other benefits before your formal offer is drafted.

It's possible to come across errors as you review the initial offer. When this happens, politely request for changes to be affected. You can contact the employer to set up a brief appointment with you to discuss the anomalies and possibly acquiesce to a counter offer.

Keep it simple and professional. For instance, you can say, "Thank you for the offer. I've reviewed the terms, and I would like to discuss the details more carefully. Please, when can we set up a time to speak?"

Be specific about the part in the offer that you want to change when you meet for the discussion. If it means writing them in a paper before the meeting, get it done to avoid missing any detail. Sometimes before big meetings I will write down my thoughts so in the heat of the conversation I don't forget or concede too easily.

On the issue of salary, provide a range that begins with the figure you'd like. For instance, if you've researched salaries for your position and determined that $5000 per month is reasonable compensation for your experience level, you could give the range of $5,000 - $7,000.

When you've successfully reached an agreement, express your gratitude and intent to sign the offer as soon as possible (that's if you're comfortable with the offer).

Dominate the Professional Image
(Nurse uniform basics + Interpersonal relationships)

"Even though your time on the job is temporary, if you do a good enough job, your work there will last forever."

Idowu Koyenikan

Getting You Equipped as You Start Off Your Nursing Career

An image is a mental picture that represents a real object; it is, more or less, an accurate likeness of person. How we view our professional self-image has an impact on our professional self-esteem. How one is perceived has an effect on performance.

Nurses all over the world are often characterized by their behavioral, physical, and professional attributes. If you asked a layman to describe the qualities of a nurse, you would get comments like, "they are neat, caring and polite individuals..." "They are beautiful hospital staffs who assist their professional superiors in a healthcare organization." These definitions of us may not be wrong. But it's not entirely true. Search for image of nurses and the most common items you see are images of nurses who are holding the hand of a frail diabetic patient, managing veterans with post-traumatic stress disorder, cradling a child who is receiving treatment for an ailment, encouraging a terminally ill patient and so on. The question is, are these all there is to say about who we are as nurses? Are these images what we leave with patients and how does it reflect on how we see ourselves? Are the characteristics of nurses limited to what they do? Does it extend to how we talk, how we look, and what we wear?

Image of Nurses to various Sections of People

Nurses are perceived differently by families, religious bodies, the media, and even other nurses themselves.

Nursing as Perceived by Religious Societies

The nursing profession comprises of various backgrounds and religions. There is no known repugnance towards the profession in every religion. However, the approach to treatments of patients varies according to beliefs and religious practices.

In most religious places, nurses are viewed as inferior to doctors. This could hurt new generation children who are deciding between options in the medical field to choose as a career choice.

For example, in most Islamic culture, it can be deduced that nurses have awareness in bringing the spiritual and cultural values in clinical practice. This includes the need to educate others to avoid pork products, gelatin, and alcoholic substances. When treating a very fervent Muslim believer, it is recommended that you look out for these listed substances in the labels of the vaccinations and medications you use.

Just like Muslims, Buddhists patients also have aversions to animal meat products. When treating a believer, ask them if they have specific dietary or treatment needs to be sure that you are in line with their culturally sensitive care.

When nursing an observant Catholic patient, be informed that the use of birth control drugs, pain management drugs during childbirth, breastfeeding, circumcision, and immunizations are all issues that are left for the discretion of the parents.

When caring for the Seventh-Day Adventist client remember that they keep the Sabbath which starts from Friday evening to Saturday evening. These clients will set aside this time for worship, family, and prayer. These clients also will not pork, shellfish, or any other unclean foods according to the Bible.

Nursing and Politics

Government policies play a significant role in the image of the nursing profession. Since Nursing is the largest medical profession in the world, it has the potential to greatly influence policy and politics on a global scale. By this, you would expect that the nursing profession should be leading the way in upgrading the healthcare system. Unfortunately, nurses have had little participation in policy that affects healthcare.

Who can blame us? A lot of governmental policies have little or no opportunity for involvement of nursing. Formal healthcare policy education in nursing is so limited that it has discouraged nursing participation in policies or politics.

Studies have shown that nurses are not provided adequate support or funding to generate the evidence needed to influence healthcare policy.

Individuals who have little or no clinical knowledge are the ones calling the shots. As a result, a lot of policies do not go in favor of a nursing practice. This has led to frustration and bitterness in the medical sector.

To be influential, nurses must begin to see themselves as professionals with the power and responsibility to influence healthcare delivery systems.

The need for policies that improve the standard of the healthcare system cannot be overemphasized. Through policy work, nurses can influence the standards of practice to ensure quality of healthcare. This extends to the allocation of funds to support healthcare delivery.

The only way the current challenges can be curbed or reduced is by encouraging political activism. This support should emanate from home – with our friends and families. Nursing schools should include healthcare policy education as a part of their curriculum. Political participation at local, state or federal level will overhaul the status quo. Someone has to be there to make our voices heard.

General Perception

One way of identifying a nurse is the dress code. Whoever said nurses must be in a white dress? Before now, healthcare organizations have let public opinions determine how they operate or appear in public. However, in recent times, many organizations have addressed this issue by changing the dress codes for their nurses.

Another generally accepted misconception is the idea of "feminine nursing." Before now, the familiar face of nursing in the media or hospital organizations is the predominant female gender in the nursing profession. This also has its effect on the image of nursing. The nursing profession is not restricted to the female populace alone.

This misconception is beginning to take a different turn as there is an increasing number of the male genders being recruited into the profession. Campaigns to draw men into the profession are now in place.

Men should begin looking at the profession the way they do other career options.

Tips on How to Resolve Conflicts

Conflicts are an inevitable aspect of human organization. The issue of compatibility is always a challenge in a setting that involves more than one individual.

Workplace conflicts, if not managed, could affect the image of the organization. Like many workplaces, it is common to see young nurses engaging in disputes that sometimes last for a long time if not carefully resolved. These conflicts could be between nursing colleagues, nurse-patients, interdepartmental, etc. these issues can be disruptive weaken your productivity.

It takes experience and skill to manage issues like this, especially when the image of the hospital is at stake.

The following are some tips on how to manage conflicts in your unit in an effective manner.

1) Maintain Calm

In the heat of the conflicts, it is common for emotions to get flared up. If you are involved in the argument, take a moment to evaluate the situation without saying a word. Are you offended? If no then calm yourself down. If yes, then calm yourself down. You have a professional image to uphold. Remember the words of the great Michelle Obama "When they go low, you go high!" It's easy to keep yell, curse, and put on a show. It is difficult to maintain your composure when someone is acting like a fool. Especially when you think you're being deprived of a particular right. Get a superior immediately. <u>Dismiss the person</u> respectfully by saying if you want to have a professional respectful conversation about the matter then meet me in the supervisor's office. If not then I do not have anything to say to you. But again, if you want to talk let's do it in front of the manager. I find that unruly staff present their concerns totally different when the supervisor is present.

When you're <u>not involved</u> in the argument or simply trying to resolve the conflict, try to maintain calm by separating the individuals affected. Discreetly separate them from the eyes of the public and away from each other. Listen to their side of the story, and when you've brought them together again, make them realize their wrongdoings. If the issue is too sensitive even for you, get an experienced staff to handle it before it gets out of control.

Note* If you are attempting to mediate tension as a *new nurse* make sure it is with staff members who report to you directly such as nurse's aides or volunteers. If you are a new nurse at a position do not attempt to mediate conflicts between seasoned nurses. That is not your responsibility, you have enough to do already. Let the nurse manager handle it.

2) Be very Attentive

When faced with a conflict, pay attention to what a person has to say and understand their perspective. This could mean, meeting directly, asking open-minded questions, and listening without interrupting.

As you listen, observe important non-verbal cues and ensure each side in the conflict understands the other's perspective. I have learned the value of accepting a person's perspective and appreciating their honesty even if it is critical of your behavior.

3) Be Diplomatic

It is possible for one side of the parties involved in the conflict to express an overwhelming point and win you over. Be cautious and stay positive. Maintain a calm demeanor throughout the conflict resolution. Remain neutral if you are mediating. Remain diplomatic if you are involved, the person may have legit reasons for contention with you and it's important that they are heard. A part of being diplomatic is also being able to admit to short comings and agree to work or grow in that under developed area. In the beginning it was hard for me to delegate tasks to older nurse's aides. I found them to be overly aggressive at my work place and didn't want to be bothered with them telling me no so I barely spoke to one in particular.

My behavior of avoidance caused us to have a strained relationship. When she brought it to my attention that I never spoke to her it was an opportunity for me to address my own personal issue. It also was an opportunity for me to apologize and move forward with a better working relationship. Being real about your good and bad is what allows for growth.

Dominate the Orientation Period

"Listen to advice and accept discipline and in the end, you will be counted among the wise." –Proverbs 19:20

Life as a New Graduate Nurse

The story below depicts a perfect instance of the ordeal new graduate nurses go through during transition. The names of the actual persons and places have been edited.

There are some traits in life that will take you far. It's not power, or strength, or wealth, it's attitude. When we graduate from nursing school sometimes we think we know all we need to be successful but that is not always the case.

Breena Dempsey was one of those gifted orientees I've supervised. She had graduated from Boston College with a GPA of 4.3. Her orientation experience was typical of most college graduates I have supervised. They start the transition with so much anxiety and nervousness until they start getting used to the idea that they can dominate the situation.

When she was formally introduced to me by my admin, she was so nervous because of what she's heard about me; 'strict, no-nonsense personality, 4 years of experience in nursing, 3 major awards from The Ohio Medical Department for Outstanding Performance in Clinical Nursing. I could tell she felt intimidated. But I'm used to that sort of introduction. I've also looked up her profile and credentials, which is what I always do when new graduate nurses are assigned to me for orientation.

The following day, she and her group walked into the hospital earlier than most of the hospital staff. They almost ran right back out of the building when they walked onto the unit. I could imagine what was going on in her mind, something like, "this wasn't how I pictured it, get me out of here!" It was a 23-bed unit, patient charts were displayed everywhere, IV poles and pumps, glucometers, precaution carts, nurses running up and down the hall, beeping sounds from the telemetry monitors showing rhythm strips. I bet she didn't know that a few weeks from then she would be getting used to all that.

She had prior clinical experience, but it was nothing compared to the reality she was facing at the Ohio Healthcare Center. Applying the skills that she had acquired during her years in school would require thorough guidance.

Two hours after she had settled in, she came up to me with some paper documents in her hands. She said, "really, paper charts? This enormous size hospital uses paper charts?" That was before we switched to electronic medical records. Just like my typical routine, I had so many workloads, and I was glad she came in when she did. I assigned some of the workload to her but not before assuring her that I'd be guiding her through it all. Her first duty was to know her dosage calculations and other medical basics.

She was very attentive as she observed how I scrupulously went through each of the patients' chart on the board. Some patients were unstable, on Cardizem drips, others heavily medicated and others in septic shock. She asked questions about every report she didn't understand. I noticed she carried a notebook and a pen with her every time. She so reminded me of myself when I was her age.

Her first task was to monitor and report the condition of a patient who had heart failure and acute respiratory distress syndrome (ARDS). When she realized that the patient was hers, she froze. During her assessment, she had forgotten to check his pedal pulses while she was assessing his temperature. The look on her face when I had to remind her to check pedal pulses showed disappointment in herself. But I quickly reassured her that it was alright. I wasn't expecting her to be perfect on her first week. Several weeks passed, and she impressed me by completing a lot of tasks. Each time we went out to get medications, I quizzed her on each of them. I gave her quite a tough time, but she understood it was to make her better.

When she came in, she was a bit nervous, overly anxious, and self-critical. She experienced difficulty trying to bond with patients or even talk to me. But after time, all that changed. She overcame those limitations and became very interactive with both her patients and nursing colleagues. She knew she had to overcome her weakness in order to assist in delivering care to her patients.

She had gained not just my confidence in her abilities, but trust from her patients and other nursing staff. She has cared for a lot of patients with a wide variety of conditions successfully ever since.

The main objectives of nursing orientation are to equip new nurses with information regarding policies, procedures, and documentation relative to their new positions. When you're fresh out of nursing school, the challenges of learning these new things plus the flow of a unit is tough.

A model regarding nursing orientation is the pairing system. An experienced nurse is paired with a relatively inexperienced nurse and supervised by an expert or nurse educator who facilitates comprehension of the nursing practice.

Preceptorship or Orientation can last for a short duration depending on the department you are working. The longest period is at the ICU, which could last for several months. My first orientation on a cardiac telemetry unit was 6 weeks however I did ask for more time because I just was not ready to be alone after that time. I was granted another 2 weeks by my unit manager.

Orientations vary according to many factors. New graduate nurses engage in practical observations and classroom studies. No matter the length of your preceptorship, there are several things you can do to make your experience as smooth as possible. Here are some things to note:

1) Orientation is overwhelming. You should be mentally ready for it. During my new graduate orientations, I was not prepared for the long classes I would have to attend after work. It was sometimes a challenge for me to stay awake at times. Definitely make sure you do not neglect sleep and try to take active notes during class. I know this seems elementary but getting up at 4 am to arrive to work, taking care of patients and then taking 2- or 3-hour classes can wear on a new nurse.

2) Nursing school teaches only the rudimentary aspects of the practice.

3) Go into the orientation with the mentality of a student.

4) Don't be afraid to ask questions. Ask relevant questions both in the classroom and on your unit.

5) Your good grades and certifications in school are essential but they do not translate to effective practice on the unit.

6) Throw away the competitive attitude you got from grade school. It's crucial you function well as a team. Letting everyone know from the beginning you are not interested in competition but are looking for opportunities to work as a team will make you a leader.

7) Learn how to delegate tasks. Don't try to do it all on your own. If you have a nurse's aide on your unit try to develop a partnership where

you can depend on each other to make the shift go smoothly. For example, I would tell my CNA I would do my own vital signs if she would assist me during a difficult dressing change. Having another pair of hands to hold a leg or arm in position can make the task so much easier.

8)   Be highly observant. It's easy to miss seemingly unimportant details that end up being significant patient information. Try to observe as much nursing care as you can.

9)   Find a good support system. Starting out as a nurse can be traumatic. Emotional trauma can affect your performance if you don't manage it. A good way of managing the stress of a new position is opening up to friends or family. Do not complain to your co-workers. Even if it looks like you are in the same boat. You are not! This will be considered highly unprofessional and most likely be reported to your supervisor even if the co-workers participate in the conversation. It is most often the new nurse who will get singled out. Trust me I know.

10)   Prioritize your learning. Try learning the most common medications on your floor – generic name, actions, side effects, etc.

11) Register your complaints when you notice that your preceptor is not good fit. If you feel like your preceptor could be more helpful in any way discuss it with your preceptor and then also bring it up during your orientation check in meetings. I would write down your thoughts before the meetings just to be sure you don't miss anything.

Personal Note: Your preceptor will make or break your orientation learning experience. You should be able to tell if you and your preceptor are going to get along within the first week. If you do not believe you two can create a good working relationship speak up immediately.
It is appropriate for you to know that your preceptor may have been mandated to take you on during the shift. It is also common for preceptors to get paid an extra dollar or two an hour when they are paired. I say this because either of those reasons could be the basis for a negative relationship and you as a new nurse should not take it personal if your preceptor is not excited about your presence.

A new nurse is another responsibility and liability to a seasoned nurse. If you have a new nurse working with you it means you have to double check your work and quadruple check theirs. As a once new nurse and also preceptor I know both sides and you have to really love to teach and share knowledge to fully embody a "preceptor."

You might want to know that I was fired from my first nursing job. That's right, I was fired. I share these details because I am your mentor and I want you to be strong where I was once weak.

I was paired with Beth. She had 11 years' experience when I arrived on the unit the first day. She let me know right away that she wanted to precept another young lady but because she didn't pass her NCLEX, she was matched with me. Let's just say Beth seemed a little annoyed from the beginning. I was a new nurse and really thought this was just the brutal honesty of the real world. I should have reported this conversation right away but again I was a new nurse and just wanted to get along with everyone.

So, for the next 8 weeks I had a miserable transition into the "real" world of nursing. I would arrive to work about an hour early every morning so I could sit in my car and cry before I walked to the unit. Nobody in my family was a nurse so even when I tried to explain what was happening to me they could not relate. Plus, others told me I only had to work 3 days a week so how bad could it really be.

I found it quite bad. Beth had a different teaching style than I learned. Her idea of preparing me for the real world was to give me the hardest patients on the unit and then watch me struggle to provide safe, competent care for 12 hours.

Literally I would walk on the unit and be told "You have the 3 hardest patients on the unit. Today you will be managing a heparin drip, a nitroglycerin drip, and an insulin drip." I want to see if you are able to make zero mistakes." My days were long; believe me, I was a new nurse and my time management skills were under developed. Sometimes Beth would help me by doing my tasks while I was in the other rooms. Although this would get me caught up I didn't really know how to provide effective because I didn't actually see anything. I also struggled to learn effectively from the written list of mistakes I had handed to me at the end of the day. As I would walk off the unit with my list of errors I felt 2 inches tall and totally incompetent as a nurse.

On my days off I would look over the list and try to research all the mistakes that were written down but the stress of the upcoming shift didn't allow me to retain much. I should have said something but I honestly just wanted to be a "good nurse" and not cause any problems.

First + Shift

One day I walked on the unit and Beth told me that we were having another meeting with the unit manager. As I walked in the room, I was told I was being terminated as I was an unsafe nurse. My manager told me that the way I struggled was unusual and she wasn't sure if nursing was a good fit for me. I left there angry that I had spent so much time learning a craft that I wasn't even good at. I went home and did what I learned to do during my 3-month orientation, I cried.

I am happy to write now the next job I landed I was paired with a great preceptor who was very patient and kind and helped me to become the nurse I am today.

I have learned a lot about being a "good nurse" one of the keys is being able to communicate effectively when things are good and when things are bad.

Your Second Home

Your workplace will become your second home, you will spend more time there than anywhere else. So, your co-workers and managers will have the opportunity to know as much about you as you want them to.

I think great work environments are cultivated and obviously take time. I want to discuss with you, the great responsibility you possess in making this happen. This is most important for you to remember your co-workers are not your friends. Your co-workers are not your family. Your co-workers are not going to sacrifice their job for yours.

I am not trying to be mean here but many new nurses like younger myself have the "I want everyone to like me complex" when starting a new position and it only brings pain to them in the end.

Remember that at the end of the day what you want people to know about you is that you are a PROFESSIONAL. You want people to understand that you are there to do a job and your service comes without drama.

You are not the one that gossips, you are not the one that openly complains. You are not the one who always has a problem. You are there to meet expectations.

Your supervisors will expect you to:

1. Have a positive, can do attitude.

2. Be a team player.

3. Ask questions when you don't know something.

4. Delegate appropriately.

5. Know and practice within your scope of practice.

6. Participate in all meetings and unit initiatives.

7. Communicate effectively.

Dominate the Patient Assignment Report

"The difference between something good and something great is attention to detail."

Charles R. Swindoll

It's time to receive your first patient assignment this is an exciting moment and you are ready! Here are the tips to ensure you are ready to take that report.

1. You arrive to work 30 minutes early.

The reason you do this is because you want to be secure that you can accomplish certain tasks such as: putting your belongings away securely, gathering your supplies for the day, setting up your work area, going to the bathroom before your shift starts and getting your report form ready so that you can take notes.

*If you have a good relationship with the charge nurse you can ask her early who she is assigning to you. Most of the time you will take over another nurse's complete assignment. So, if she says you will take over Michelle's patients then you can get started researching those patients

before you are even clocked in. There may be some who don't agree to starting work before being clocked in but remember you are not performing any tasks or providing care. Once you get a finalized assignment you can do what I call my *Pre-Report Pass.* This means going into each room and quickly dialoging with the client.

2. Pre-Report Pass

I would say "Hello, my name is Regina. How would you like me to address you? Ok Mr. Smith, I will be your registered nurse for the next shift I begin at 7:30 pm. I will be the one to give your medications and do your nursing treatments I really can provide all your nursing care but I have help. I am working with Tiffany, she is the nurse's aide. She will be assisting me.

Tiffany is here to get your meals, take you to the restroom and help you with your personal care. I just wanted to stick my head in and take a look at you before I receive report. I will be back in about 20 minutes to do a complete assessment." When I return is there anything I can bring you?"

Make sure to write down the patient's requests. Don't trust your brain to remember because you will be learning a lot of information in the next few minutes.

(This will be the close of the "*Pre-Report Pass*")

Notes about the "*Pre-Report Pass*"

*When you introduce yourself also quickly orient the patient to the other staff if possible so they can make choices about who to call based off their needs. If a client understands that there is another staff responsible for making the bed, they will not call the licensed nurse to do the task. A well-informed patient can make the best decision, so let's empower our patients with knowledge!

Another pre-report task you should try to accomplish is reading the doctor's progress notes on the client. What is the last note the doctor wrote? Read it. This will help you to know the patient's condition. Is the patient getting better or worse?

If you have access to the chart review the lab values and treatment orders that are needed. All of this information is very helpful to have before accepting the client. The *Pre-Report* pass should be done in about 10 minutes for each client. This will be a goal time for you to reach it will not happen right away.

If you follow this technique you will go into the patient handoff report with a clear vision of who you are assigned to care for. When you sit down to take report with your report form you will gather all the necessary information to effectively care for the client. See the report form below.

This is a sample view of my report form. Feel free to make your own.

RM #		RM #	
NAME:		NAME:	
AGE:	SEX:	AGE:	SEX:
ISO:	TELE:	ISO:	TELE:
DX:		DX:	
HX:		HX:	
ALLERGIES:		ALLERGIES:	
CODE STATUS:		CODE STATUS:	
ACCU CHECKS:		ACCU CHECKS:	
DIET:		DIET:	
MD:		MD:	
ACTIVITY:		ACTIVITY:	
IV ACCESS:		IV ACCESS:	
NEURO:		NEURO:	
CARDIO:		CARDIO:	
RESP:		RESP:	

3. Declining a Patient Assignment

It's rare for a patient assignment to be declined.

This is because the decision to refuse a patient assignment is a difficult one. Finding yourself in a predicament where a patient's health is at stake and the consequences of losing your employment are dangling in front of you, it can become challenging to make this decision.

The sole purpose of refusing a patient assignment is for safety reasons.

It takes discretion and knowledge to determine when it is proper to decline a patient assignment and it also takes courage to speak up when patient safety is compromised.

The following are some reasons why a patient assignment may be rejected:

> *Excess patients*

In some cases, patient assignments are declined because the facility lacks space to accommodate new intakes. This can be very awkward, especially in cases of emergency. There may be safe nurse patient ratios that need to be maintained which would be a legit reason to refuse any new admissions.

> *Being too fatigued*

Working several hours without a break could exhaust the workforce physically. If you feel too tired it is probably best to not even come in to work rather than come in mentally compromised and cause patient harm.

> *Lack of qualification or training*

Some nurses may lack the experience to care for complicated medical cases. The wisest decision is to assign the complex client to an experienced nurse.

> *Receiving patient without communication or hand off report*

Agreeing to care for a patient who you know nothing about is a dangerous assignment that could lead to patient harm. It is necessary to know important medical details before agreeing to care for a patient.

> *Receiving two patients with similar last names.*

There is no reason for a nurse to have two patients with the same last names. For example, Carol Brown and James Brown. This puts the nurse under an unnecessary strain to avoid mixing up treatments and/or medications. As a new nurse do not let this happen to you.

Dominate the Patient Introduction

"It's not ideas, nor visions, nor tools that truly mater in therapy. If you debrief patients at the end of therapy about the process, what do they remember? Never the ideas – it's always the relationship."

Irvin D. Yalom

Establishing Trust through Your Introduction

As rewarding and fulfilling as caring for patients can be, it is also sometimes emotionally and physically draining. Nurses is a combination of two professions – patient care and customer service. Maintaining a professional, courteous interpersonal relationship can be daunting. It can also prove useful in a patient's overall health and well-being.

It is very essential to establish a healthy nurse-patient relationship. It can be the major difference in determining the pace of your patient's recovery. You should greet the patient by name, make eye contact, and display confidence and expertise.

You can engage your patient in a conversation centering on your schedules for the shift. Explain everything they will be doing and review the plan of care, making sure to involve them in decision making where possible. Also, have in mind that maintaining patient privacy is essential.

For some patients, touch is a way to demonstrate compassion and caring, but you should be aware of their personal boundaries. Use your discretion.

Remaining culturally sensitive is also important, providing handouts and patient information in a patient's language should be offered, as well as an interpreter if required. These vital items help to develop trust and open lines of communication.

How Does Trust and Communication Aid Patients?

At the initial stage, when patients seek health care or are hospitalized, most of them are not familiar with the process and what to expect. They may be nervous about what's to come and not understand the medical terms being spoken. Hearing medical terminologies may be like a foreign language. They could be overwhelmed with the feeling of helplessness which will likely lead to frustration and resistance to learning.

A healthy nurse-patient relationship, if established from the onset, will help the patient feel more at ease. And instead of the feeling of frustration, they will open up and participate in the care process.

Creating an Impression

When you are just meeting a patient for the first time, create an air of trust. It doesn't take rocket science. Your appearance and manner of approach is an excellent way to create an impression that will set off a good relationship.

Sometimes when some nurses complain that a patient is "difficult," if you really listen to what they are saying, you will understand that they are not actually difficult but have an unmet need.

Some people say it takes approximately 15 seconds to make a lasting impression and the rest of your life to undo it. The following are basic etiquettes you can execute to ensure your first impression is a good one:

As useful as communication skills are in interpersonal relationships, it's not the only factor needed to ensure nurses successfully interact or work with patients. Trust is required to establish a relationship between the nurse and the patient.

Although there are many other ways your role as a nurse could be communicated to patients, professional greetings are a powerful way to show your role in the care of the patient. The professional introduction also makes definite the nurse's accountability to the patient. It brings to light, the nurse's knowledge and professionalism, helping to emphasize nurses' responsibilities which is often not well understood by the general public.

Begin by keeping it simple:

Your first words should express some form of appreciation or compliments, depending on the context of your dialogue. Make it simple and polite, for instance, if you are just meeting for the first time and you don't have their name, you can say, "Good morning, my name is James, I'm a Registered Nurse, it is nice to meet you."

When you begin with statements like that, establish eye contact and wait for them to respond.

Posture:

When you approach your patient, walk with an air of vigor and vitality. Don't drag your feet as you walk.

Don't lean on structures when you start off your conversation. As a nurse you represent health, therefore personify it in your movement and posture.

Groom your hair:

Appearance also matters. You should reflect impeccable grooming. Don't walk in with your hair wet or with your hair falling unto your face. Nervous and distracting gestures such as touching and scratching your scalp should also be avoided.

Your footwear:

Your physical features from the floor up should be impeccable. Don't walk into the room with dusty and worn-out shoes. They'll detract from your professional image. If you work in any healthcare setting your shoes are at risk for becoming soiled and visibly dirty. Make it a habit to wash your shoes or buy new ones regularly.

Dominate the Shift Assignment

"Until we can manage time, we can manage nothing else."

Peter F. Drucker

Now that you have your client reports you are able to act fully as the nurse on duty. Most of your colleagues will quickly run off to look at their patients but because you arrived early and know who they are and what they are doing you can engage yourself in other important tasks.

During this time, you are to take a look at your "*Hourly Task Manager*" for each client. (A sample of this form is found on the following page).

You will head to the client's chart and note medication and treatment times. You do not need to write down each medication name, just note the time that the task should be accomplished. Writing them down on this form will allow you to see your day's activities at a glance. This will also allow you to see if you will have any free time. If so, let a co-worker know you will be able to assist them if needed during that time. This step may take up to 20 minutes but it will guide you throughout the rest of the shift.

Remember you are a team leader, organization makes that possible.

(*This is a form I created in Microsoft word.)

Sample Hourly Task Manager

RM #	102- J, Brown	105 K, Daniels
800	Prepare Am Meds	Needs Pain Meds Do Assessment
900	Assess + Document	Document
1000	PO Med Due	Chart
1100	Check blood sugar Give insulin, Snack	IV antibiotic due Chart
1200	Write Progress Note	
1300		Assess pain give meds
1400	Ambulate 12 ft	Wound dressing change
1500	Hang New IV fluids Meds Due	Document
1600		PO Meds due
1700	Check Bld sugar	
1800	Final Round Document	Post NPO after Midnight sign/ Final round
IVF	NS @ 100 ml/hr	None
TO DO	TESTS/PROCEDURES/LABS	TESTS/PROCEDURES/LABS
	Draw pm labs Chest x-ray in am	Call OR to see if surgery time scheduled

62

During your shift you will do a mandatory minimum of "5 Passes" into your patient's room. Some facilities require their nurses to be in the client's room every hour. If you do more excellent that is awesome but you must do these 5. The 5 Passes are the:

1. The Pre-report Pass - This is the first introduction of who you are and the opportunity to see if the client has any imminent needs that you can address when you return or the reporting nurse should address before giving the client over to you.

2. The Second Hello and Assessment Pass - This is the opportunity when you return to the room to spend more time with the client and also do your first complete assessment. You should also make sure the client has used the bathroom and has a full pitcher of water for when you return.

3. The Medication Pass - This is the opportunity that you are able to come into the room with the priority focus of effectively administering medications. You are also able to do your client education and give important medications. Because you have been in the room at least twice the client should have less reason to disrupt this process. Remember your medication pass does not end until all of the medications have been properly documented.

4. The Treatment Pass - The focus of this visit is to complete any treatments that are due. This includes ambulation activities, incentive spirometry, wound dressing changes, IV dressing changes or site changes. Any treatments that you are to do or if you can help out the on-coming nurse by doing them early, this is the time. Remember if you are doing anything that might cause pain, medicate your clients about 30 minutes to 1 hour beforehand.

5. The Goodbye Pass - This pass is necessary as it provides closure to the client that his excellent nurse will be departing. Always thank the client for allowing you to provide care and if you know the oncoming nurse tell the client her name and something you like about her. This will make the client feel more comfortable with the transition and your soft introduction may serve as his/her Pre-report Pass if they do not do one.

*Your first shifts will be challenging but you will be more prepared if you have this game plan.

Work Routines

Work routine varies according to the healthcare organization. Shifts are allotted based on the size of the facility.

Most new graduate nurses work a 12-hour shift. A good number of new nurses also work multiple shifts or extra shifts.

Working overtime could pose problems for patients and nurses. Common challenges such as burn out, medication errors, occupational injuries, and job dissatisfaction are associated with working overtime. This is one of the reasons why compulsory overtime is restricted by law in most states in the USA. Individuals who usually fall victim to such hospital policies are the new nurses.

Working Night Shifts

Experienced nurses in most healthcare systems have the advantage of getting the shifts they want, this leaves the new nurses to work uncomfortable routines.

If you are one of those nurses that dread night-shift, you shouldn't be. Working night shifts also has its perks. You will come to prefer it if you learn how to maximize your time and use the routine to your advantage.

Not saying that the night shifts doesn't have its challenges, especially for new nurses or nurses who are new to the shift, but there are some benefits too.

Benefits of Working Nights

✓ High demand for Night Shift Nurses: A lot of hospitals place top priorities for night shift nurses. It's not so much as a fancy choice, but it is an opportunity one should embrace in this recession. I only worked night shifts because it allowed me to have amazing opportunities.

✓ The monetary advantage: Night shifts fall under less popular work routine, but there's a pay differential that accompanies night shift routines.

✓ Less Distractions: Working night shifts give you time to concentrate on your patient care. Emergency cases are higher during the day, that always leave hospital staffs running around from Intensive Care Units to the OR and giving little time to other patients. You also have less people on the unit in terms of management, visitors, and ancillary staff. This means more work space, less new orders for your patients, and more time to do things such as treatments or investigate progress.

✓ You have your alone time: You enjoy autonomy and opportunity to learn at your own pace. At many of the hospitals I worked at new graduates started on night shifts once off orientation for this reason.

Common Risks Associated with Night-Shift Nurses

Night shift nurses also face challenges during or after their routines. Post-work stress is majorly the hazards that accompany night-shift routines.

Ever heard the term "nocturnal humans?" well, that's a rare case. Evading sleep can impede your natural clock, which can affect your body in the form of insomnia, weight gain, and heart disease.

Night shifts also affect your social life and could alter your social circle.

How to Adapt Successfully to Night-Shift Nursing

I. Every Nurse adapts differently. Our bodies are different. Each person has a biological clock ticking away inside of their brain, and a bunch of tiny biological clocks in the entire body. Unlike a regular clock, not every person's biological clock keeps the same time or rotate at the same pace.

You must have heard someone say, "I'm not a morning person." This is the reason. Some people function better in the night than at morning and vice versa.

Natural early risers tend to have a tough time adjusting to night-shift nursing compared to others.

II. Don't skip any chance you get to sleep or have a nap. Get at least 6 – 8 hours of uninterrupted sleep within a 24-hour period. You can get this done by shutting down electronic gadgets and letting those around you know not to disturb. Avoid taking caffeine 4 hours prior to your bedtime. Also limit activity and exercise before going to sleep.

It's important for your mental well-being that you give the body adequate rest to avoid breakdown. If you're the type that doesn't sleep easily, create a conducive environment for it. Blackout curtains, melatonin or use a facemask if you have to.

III.   Keep your family or roommates in the loop about the recent change in your schedule. This will ensure that there are no surprises or intrusion that might affect your routine and nap time.

IV.   Be on the lookout for the unexpected while on duty. Besides the fact that daytime shifts are known for a lot of activities, it is also possible to have emergency situations on night shift too. Ensure you understand the procedures and who to call or consult for guidance or assistance.

V.   Study your own medications thoroughly to know every detail, such as side effects, prescription, age limits, contents, etc. Also, avoid drugs that could impair your alertness and performance on duty.

VI.   Don't take the steering wheel or attempt to work when you are drowsy. Drowsiness can blur your vision and alter your judgment or alertness

VII.   Your brain needs to be active. Therefore, you need to take scheduled breaks once in a while. The job can be so engaging and exciting that you could feel tempted to skip you break times. But remember, your mental health is also for the benefit of your patient, your job, and yourself.
There are several hospitals that provide a separate space or room for staffs to take naps during breaks. However, set an alarm to ensure you don't oversleep.

VIII.   Eat well and stay hydrated. Skipping meals may also have a disadvantage on the body system, which could affect your performance on duty. Sometimes, activities pile up on some shifts prompting you to be on your feet for most of the time. Drink at least 8 glasses of water every day to stay hydrated. Drinking at least 24 ounces in a 12hour shift can keep you refreshed.

Gastrointestinal problems like bloating, constipation, nausea, etc. occurs as a result of skipping dinner or breakfast.

IX.   If you discover that you are continually fatigued even after a good rest, talk to a doctor.

X.   Sometime, you will discover that there is no activity in your unit. During such dormant periods, stay productive. You can use such time to complete other tasks that you've put on hold. Finish up your documentations. Staying busy will help you stay alert.

This could be different when you work in the ER or the Labor and Delivery Unit, where babies arrive on their own timetable.

XI.   Maintain excellent communication at shift transitions. Ask the day-shifts nurses a lot of questions to ensure you have accurate details. Patients and their family may be unreliable when trying to get feedback for your report. This will help you avoid any negative surprises regarding the health status of your patients.

XII.   Build rapport with your fellow night shift nurses. Engaging in a professional conversation with them will keep you alert, especially during dormant periods.

Also, you can learn a thing or two while chatting with experienced nurses.

Dealing with The Feeling of Incompetency

New nurses tend to develop an insecurity complex in the first few weeks of service. Transitioning into the real practice could have that effect, but it's your responsibility resist such mindset.

To stop feeling incompetent as a nurse, the first step is to believe in yourself. <u>You Can, You Will, You Must Dominate Your Shift!</u> Understand that the process takes time and requires getting used to.

As you adapt to your new career and observe your experienced colleagues don't be afraid of asking questions.

New graduate nurses often make common mistakes like giving medications late, entering the wrong assessment into reports, and so on. But don't let the feeling you get from making these errors overwhelm you. You've prepared well for this, finished your nursing school, beat the NCLEX, and you will overcome this nursing practice – it only takes consistency and time.

Understand that you still have more mistakes to make in your journey to excellence in your career.

Ask most new nurses in their first 6 months of practice how they are managing, and you will notice they have the following things in common:

- The Feeling of incompetence, stress, and worry that they are *always doing the wrong thing*.
- The fear of asking too many questions.
- Having problems with time management and difficulties managing various tasks at once.
- Feeling inefficient or unfit to handle a task, thereby wasting precious time.
- Proficiency in handling medications and confusing one prescription with the other.

To say you're not alone is an understatement.

What to do?

Surviving your first two years as a nurse without undermining your professional skills and potential abilities requires positive practical steps

1) **Introduce yourself to everyone** - Register your person in every circle or department you find yourself. Don't hide behind the curtains. Introduce yourself to everyone – the janitors, reception staff, clinical assistants, colleagues, and superior officials.

   Letting people know who you are in a new place creates an opportunity for friendship, interactions with more experienced staffs, etc.

   Sometimes, all it takes to start a good relationship is just "hello, my name is ...., it's nice to meet you." Be nice. Be willing to learn from everyone. You are new people are probably wondering who you are, too.

   The sooner you introduce yourself, the easier it becomes to feel more comfortable with your new unit. Get on to it and get over with it! Most people will warmly welcome you as you introduce yourself and may even offer to help before you ask.

2) **Continuous Practice makes the difference** - It's usual to start off with a positive attitude and turn a new leaf all of a sudden. Work stress could have that effect on you.

   If you've connected well with your patients probably by listening to them, smiling each time you drop in to check on them, please continue with that.

3) **Start with what you know** - Start with the things you are good at and build from there. Care for your patients as you would your loved ones. Speak to them in the language they will understand. Breaking down medical terms and explaining what the doctor has said using words they understand foster your relationship with them.

4) **Have a Go-to crew** - This is not the time to play lone wolf. You need a reliable team or support group to get you through some difficult situations that are beyond you.

   As you start to make acquaintances on the unit, you will inevitably meet people with whom you "click" with right away. Try to find at least one nurse, one doctor, and another team member (maybe a charge nurse) who are most eager to guide you. Think of them as mentors and utilize them!

You'll not only grow an active personal and professional bond with them but, you'll become a much stronger nurse as you proactively seek guidance throughout your first two years.

5) **Have the right tools** - Equipment which allows you to look good and perform the job, even if you don't really know what you're doing just yet.

6) **Don't get personal** - As a new nurse, learn to keep things professional as much as possible. It's very likely for doctors, nurses, patients, and other hospital staffs to take their frustrations out on you sometimes.

If anyone makes a shift difficult for you, react differently. Maturity has nothing to do with age or intelligence. Prove that you're more professional by the way you handle the matter. Don't give anyone the avenue to make their problems yours.

7) **Act Confident** - Even when you are terrified, <u>fake it</u> and act confident. Keep an open mind while at it. A wise person said "*fake it until you make it!*"

If you're asked to complete a task you're new to, don't decline the opportunity to do it. Be open to new experiences but spend time researching about the new tasks. Don't be afraid to questions and even seek an experienced nurse to be present to guide you. Explain to the patient that the two of you will be doing the task together. Some might think that will cause distress but the patient may be happy to know that double the care is being provided to make sure the procedure goes smoothly.

8) **Keep a Straight Face** - Every day in your routine, you will come across different people with different sort of reactions and opinions - some horrible, incredible, peculiar and some downright ridiculous. You need to develop a poker face. Keep a straight face and not give too much away to maintain your composure and stay dignified.

Evidently, nurses have the best poker faces in the business. You will see it all as a new nurse – organs prolapsing from not-so-correct anatomical locations, obscene tattoos on decrepit patients, explosive diarrhea, belligerent little woman, mentally challenged patients, addicts, ex-convicts escorted by law enforcement officers, and the list go on. You will have patient's say very strange things, ask you questions that will baffle your clinical know-how, or sometimes code and die in front of you. And through it all, you learn to keep a poker face.

Watch your experienced colleagues and observe how they cope with various feedbacks. Having a poker face enables you to remain professional and unbiased. It might take time to master, but you will get better at it with time.

9) **Listen to the Doctor's Rounds** - Get used to observing the doctors when they make assessments and speak about the patient's care evaluations. You may have to introduce yourself first so that you can have the opportunity to ask necessary questions. I usually don't ask question but just hang out looking busy but there might be a rare occasion you have a friendly relationship with a doctor and can do so.

This tip is very essential for any new graduate nurses, most of what they are saying may not make 100% sense at first, but will in due time.

10)   **Express yourself** - Communicating like a professional nurse is an art that takes some time to master. It's not in the school curriculum - it's a skill you honestly have to learn in practice. You will eventually learn to give the report to colleagues but, until you find a style and flow that works for you, "SBAR" is a good place to start.

Try as much as you can to avoid using abbreviations when talking to persons who lack clinical knowledge. Always explain acronyms when educating your patients. You are not trying to impress your patients. Very often, you see a doctor or nurses say things to their patients like, "we are just going to do a CBC, BMP, and type and screen for now" while the patient smiles and nods ignorantly.

It's essential to think about more effective ways to communicate with patients. For instance, say, "we are going to draw some blood out of that IV line so the team can assess your levels. We'll be evaluating your blood count, like red and white blood cells, and your chemistry profile, like your electrolyte levels. We will also confirm your blood type in case you need a blood transfusion in the future." This example of a breakdown makes it easier for your patients and their family members to understand.

How to Feel Better About Awkward Experiences as a New Nurse

Adjusting into professional practice as a nurse takes time. You have to get used to embarrassing situations and not let them weigh you down emotionally. This may be easier said than done.

Instances:

If it's discovered that a patient in your care has just disappeared, leaving you with no clue of their whereabouts.

The feeling of awkwardness will instantly take the place of curiosity. This might affect your performance for a while, especially if you're not used to dealing with embarrassing situations in public places.

You need to develop the critical thinking skills to work out potential places your patient could be as there is really only really a handful of locations they are.

Ask yourself questions like –

- "Is he/she an alcoholic/drug abuser/cigarette smoker and looking for the substance?" (This is likely because addicts are accustomed to being fidgety and edgy when they are relapsing).
- "Does he/she have a mental related problem?" (Patients with mental problems act unusual)
- "Is he/she looking for a doctor?" (Another possible reason why he/she may want to leave his ward).
- "Is he/she going out for fresh air?" (Some patients get claustrophobic when left in a secluded space for a long time).
- Is she/he looking for a vending machine to go off the prescribed diet? (Some clients do not like hospital food and just want to have a Snickers.)
- Is she/he looking for a cellphone charger?

Critical questions like this will help you assess the possible outcome or solution. No wonder it is referred to as 'critical thinking.' The faster you start analyzing the "why," the easier nursing will become, and the more you will enjoy that aspect of the profession.

Another embarrassing situation that new nurses often find themselves in is:

Pressing the Code or Blue or Emergency button while trying to turn off the patient call bell.

This can be very hilarious, but not to the nurse who did it. But you can look at the brighter side of it. Just assume that you have used the opportunity to learn the functions of each button. You can wittingly turn the jokes on your nursing colleagues. Make them believe it was a prank call to keep everyone on their toes. Sometimes you have to just laugh at yourself and that's ok.

Are you Fearful of asking too many questions as a new nurse?

The idea of not asking too many questions in order not to lose your professional grandeur is common to new nurses. No good teacher gets offended by questions, no matter how repetitive they are. However, it could get awkward in a tense situation. You should use your discretion. Asking a doctor or your senior colleagues questions at a time when you should be quiet and observant is one way of finding yourself on the road to "Awkward-Ville."

Before you ask some questions, take a few seconds to see if you can find the answer on your own first.

Here are some tips on finding the answer for yourself as a new nurse:

- Examine the doctor's notes in your patient's file to find the plan. If something doesn't look right, get to the lab and check CT/x-ray/MRI/US results for answers.

- While you're checking the results of any tests/lab reports/surgery information, jump to the conclusion section of the report which is usually at the bottom page, where you will find some golden information on what's going on with your patient. It's legibly typed, so you don't have issues trying to make out the handwriting.

- Also, look up the hospital policy about the subject or procedure you're not sure about. There are policies for everything. Make sure you are using the search option effectively. ("Ctrl + F" is a great keyboard shortcut to find the exact words you're looking for in a long piece of text).

Remember, all nurses before you had a similar experience, so you don't have to feel alone when you're in the same situation.

Accept the fact that you are new and be teachable. Start picking the brain of these nurses who you admire, but try working a few things out on your own.

Asking questions and bouncing ideas off somebody can make sure you're on the right track while being correct can give you a big shot of confidence.

Before you call The Doctor

There are certain awkward situations you can avoid. Ensure you've straightened things out on your end before calling the doctor. Don't give patients and their family members the notion that you are helpless.

Here are a few things you can do;

- Ensure you have clarified orders, admitted patients with the paper works appropriately done.
- Obtain pain relief materials and straighten out your next plan
- Check to identify the right doctor to call.
- Find out the urgency of the case to give accurate feedback to the doctor
- Have pertinent information in front of you like client's chart and medication record.

New nurses and even experienced ones also feel anxious when speaking to the doctor, particularly when the person answering is also agitated. Prepare a list, be prepared, and ask questions.

Make adequate preparations to have a well-detailed presentation. This will save you the stress of running around in case of insufficient data or material.

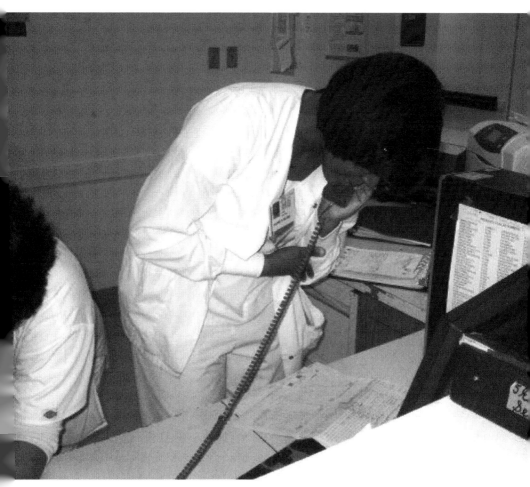

Myself as a new graduate, speaking to the doctor and looking directly at the client's orders so I could be prepared to answer any question. – Washington, DC 2009

TIME MANAGEMENT

Juggling all the tasks and responsibilities in your schedule, and having to manage your personal life can be very chaotic if you're new to the experience.

You probably listed time management as one of your skills, but the real deal is having to confront the actual experience will test you.

Great nurses weren't made overnight. There are strategies to time management that new nurses can learn. Effectively managing your time will make the transition easier to adjust to. The following are some key strategies you should learn how to inculcate into your routine:

1) **Set Your Priorities Right** - This strategy takes getting used to. It is a common subject that appears on the NCLEX. Learn how to prioritize your tasks in order to manage the stress that accompanies the multiplicities efficiently. The complexity of medical conditions varies considerably, and most of them won't fit within the parameters you outline.

   To understand the order of importance in each task and how to prioritize them, you should be able to answer the following questions:

   - What's more important for the patient I'm caring for?
   - What's the first thing you should do and why?
   - Is there a consequence if you don't act now? What could happen?
   - Which task is more important, and why?

   Answering these questions will help you find the value of each task and the costs of decision making. You can engage this exercise with other nurses to get a second opinion. Two heads are better than one after all. Critical thinking skills are effectively achieved when there are more people involved.

2) **Recognize the Value of Adaptability and Patience** - Some of the qualities of healthcare professionals are patience and level-headedness in the face of chaos and frightening situations.

   No matter how peaceful the environment looks, there is always the issue of fears and uncertainties buried in every case you handle. In addition to that, are criticisms from the public, challenges you face working with other people and so on.

   In as much as setting priorities and having a plan are vital tactics to get through your day, you also need to have patience and be adaptable to the changing circumstances you are likely to come across.

   As part of your duties as a nurse, confronting, the unknown is inevitable. If you're exhausted because it took you a long time to complete a task, got often interrupted during your shift, or had to deal with situations that took you out of your zone, it's okay. Mental exhaustion doesn't get you anywhere, so sometimes, it's best to embrace the fact that your carefully planned shift is heading in an alternative direction. Remember your role, struggle to get it back where it needs to be, and don't dwell on the unplanned events.

3) **Learn to cluster care** - Since you're new to the experience, it's normal for you to work at a slower pace compared to your more experienced colleagues. It's a common phenomenon in every field of work. There is so much value in doing a task over and over again. The more you do it, the more experience you gain at it and the quicker you become, consequently, freeing up time for other tasks.

   As you gain more experience repeating specific tasks, the more you'll be able to anticipate your next move and a patient's need. You can start clustering things together as you go.

   What future tasks around you can you complete before you have to run across the unit twice? How many immediate needs can you address before handling the responsibilities that can wait till the end of your shift?

   Be proactive. Always think about your next move, keeping the big picture in mind.

4) **Take A Break When You Need It** - It's essential to take a break to collect your thoughts no matter how briefly. You are not a robot. A 5 minutes recess will do you a lot of good, especially when you've been busy for too long. Drink some water to rehydrate, reassemble your thought process, and hop back into your shift. As a nurse, it's usual to run into a long period of active engagement that keeps you standing on your feet for a long time. Go to the restroom, take a break to avoid fatigue, burnout, or any medical condition.

Nutritional Tips for New Nurses

Working as a new nurse can be very tough. Distractions and tasks, you've been assigned to do can keep you starving for the entire shift. Short breaks might not be enough to give attention to your nutritional needs.

Remember, you can only give what you have. You can't function well in your shift if your body system is deprived of essential nutrients.

You've learned how to look your best. Nice clothes, moderate makeup, and fashion accessories can only go as far as you feel and look physically.

An entire week can be occupied with a busy schedule, but don' subscribe to the idea that you will only eat when you are hungry. Your enthusiasm for the job could deny you the appetite to nourish your body system. It's challenging to have three square meals on a typically busy work routine.

According to research by the Federal Agency for Healthcare Research and Quality, nurses regularly miss meals to care for patients. As a result, most nurses resort to snacks during meal breaks. High-calorie items are therefore consumed in enormous amount as a result. What this means for you is putting on an additional 10 to 20 pounds during the first two years of being a nurse if you are not careful.

Tips for Healthy Eating

It is crucial for your body system that you revitalize by eating well-nourished meals. Most options don't take much time to prepare. Healthy eating leads to better weight management and improved performance at work.

1) **Avoid skipping meals** - Skipping mealtimes affects your digestive setting in such a way that it begins to rely on the little energy reserve you have. Changes like fatigue, drop of glucose level, loss of concentration, and irritable feeling begins to surface. The brain requires glucose to function. When a certain period elapses, the body uses the protein content in the body. As the fasting progresses, the body resorts to using fats (ketone content) to preserve the remaining protein. Ketosis could be the next impact if the fasting continues. Ketosis is a metabolic state in which the body produces ketones to be used as fuel by some internal organs so that glycogen can be reserved for other organs in the body. When ketosis takes effect, the body begins to experience nausea, low blood pressure, and fatigue.

   This can affect your performance on your shifts. Another problem that can result from skipping a meal is the sudden blood glucose reaction; leading to increased triglyceride content. This can also lead to weight gain.

   It's also recommended that you divide your nutrient fill over the course of the day instead of taking it all in a single course.

2) **Limit your intake of caffeine content** - It is common for night shift workers to take coffee which has caffeine contents to stay alert. Even energy drinks such as Rock-Star or Red-Bull are common for nurses to use. However too much caffeine can lead to insomnia, cardiac problems, and other medical conditions. One of the first signs of a caffeine abuse is chest palpitations.

3) **Stay hydrated** - For essential bowel function, blood circulation and regulation of body temperature, it is important to hydrate often. When the body suffers dehydration, the body can get also become fatigued which can lead to temperature issues and heart problems.

   It can really be surprising how unhealthy nurses are due to work related stressors. Drink at least 8 cups of water regularly to cleanse your body system and hydrate the body.

4) **Take your own meals or snacks to night shifts** - You can relax and eat your prepared meal at break time.

5) **Relax When Eating** - Some shifts can be full of activities but take your time to relax when eating your meal to avoid getting indigestion. Ensure you're in relaxed mode before having your meal to aid proper digestion. Your patients need you refreshed and healthy.

6) **Plan your mealtime** - Understand your work schedule and take some time to plan your mealtime. Any day you choose to eat at the cafeteria or restaurant close to your facility, endeavor to read their menu before ordering. There may be a healthy option that you didn't expect to be available.

7. **Schedule your routine mealtimes** - Few weeks into the job, you should be able to understand the work routine. Sort out your task priorities and stick to a particular schedule using your *Hourly Task Manager* form.

8. **Limit your consumption of snack** - Nurses are notorious for organizing potlucks. We love to bring in baked goods to please the staff. Try as much as you can to resist the temptation to eat just any snacks. If you are going to eat snacks, choose a more nutritious snack like crackers, wheat chips, granola, etc. you can find some of these in a vending machine. If possible abstain from processed foods as a regular snack.

9. **Engage in regular exercise** - A good meal plan will not be complete without regular exercises to regulate your body metabolism. It also helps your digestive system, blood circulation, mental alertness, and muscular structure.

Hit the gym when you can or run around your neighborhood when you get the chance to.

Don't let the fact that you are too busy cause you to neglect this vital information.

Dominate Speaking to the Manager, Doctor or Anyone Else

"Ambition is the path to success. Persistence is the vehicle you arrive in."

Bill Bradley

Improving Interpersonal Skills Relevant to Your Work Ethics

Effective communication skills will help you as you transition into full-time practice. Besides reducing the discomfort associated with joining an establishment, maintaining proper communication reflects positively on your professional contribution. Look at it this way, you're one of the many screws that keep that establishment together. A strong communication network between you and your unit, doctors, and managers will have a positive impact on the organization's image and productivity.

In our workplace, we should endeavor to remediate bad communication because it undercuts our ability to be efficient. If you look up various successful organizations, you will discover that employees in such settings communicate well, consequently increasing productivity.

Everyone yearns to be heard. That's the reason behind so many social media platforms. At the workplace, it is natural to exercise those characteristics. We care about opinions of our coworkers, managers, doctors, etc.

In your two years of nursing, try to connect and communicate effectively with coworkers, doctors, and members of your management team. Don't crawl back to your shell when experiencing any setback. Keep practicing and developing your communication skills.

You may be a new employee, but your contributions are substantial. Nurses are on the frontlines of care, creating effective nurse-patient communication that leads to a positive experience.

A good interpersonal relationship with your colleagues and superior staffs will create a healthy structure.

WHAT DOES A HEALTHY NURSE-PATIENT COMMUNICATION LOOK LIKE?

The nursing profession is a career dedicated to serving the needs of our patients. This requires various tactics, including patient education. A healthy nurse-patient communication ensures that care is given smoothly without any secondary complications

Some of these communication strategies are either to foster an interpersonal relationship or ensure a patient cooperates.

1) **Non-Verbal Approach** - You can pass on a message to an audience without making a sound. Nurses use this skill when words do not apply in the context or a fundamental approach to achieve result. Non-verbal communication is a practical skill that establishes a connection between the nurse and the patients.

   This approach includes making eye contacts, using body languages, or merely smiling at the patient as a way of bonding with them. Your posture can also be interpreted by the patient to mean something. In some cases where patients can't speak because they are not fully conscious or using a respirator, non-verbal communications is a highly effective way of connecting to the patient.

2) **Active listening** - Ever been in a situation where you are talking to someone while he's also talking back at the same time? There's no communication in such an instance. Communication is reached when the message is actually passed across. This is why listening is an effective way of reaching an understanding.

   Some patients want to be listened to. While everyone is busy telling them, what might be wrong with them, or the cause and suggestive solutions to their predicaments, they just want someone who can actively listen (not pretend to listen). You may be the expert, but the patient is the one having the aches and pains. Perhaps their body is reacting differently to the intravenous medication administered to them.

Listen to understand; <u>don't be in a hurry to respond</u>. It's a good principle that creates the opportunity to win the heart of your patient. You could nod your head in response while you maintain a relaxed posture.

Being attentive is vital to the overall patient experience. Frequent check-in on your patients reduces both physical and emotional distress.

An attentive nurse understands a patient even more than most of their family members. You know their worries, fears and as a result, alleviate these concerns, leading to progress in their health status.

3) **Showing Compassion** - Sympathy often tells in our posture, expressions, and even actions. Being hospitalized is sad and deserving of compassion. No one comes to the hospital for vacations. Show respect and compassion when treating your patients.

   This has often proven to be an effective way of getting patients (even the difficult ones) to cooperate.

4) **Verbal Communications** - Unlike the non-verbal skill, here you use words to pass your message across. It is a very vital approach as a lot can be communicated using words. Talk to your patients in clear, complete sentences without raising your tone.

5) **Interpersonal Relationship** - There's a need to establish trust and cooperation of your patients. Some nurses are so good at this that their organizations can't afford to lose them.

   Learn how to show compassion, care, and kindness when you are reaching out to your patient. This will help the patient feel accepted and willing to heed instructions relevant to their care.

6) **Learn to keep your words** - Don't make promises you can't keep. So often, in our zeal to make the patients feel hopeful, we say things they want to hear. Be mindful of the promises you make to your patients.

   Take their concerns seriously but always keep your word. This will establish the trust they have in you.

7) **Patient education** - This is a crucial aspect of nursing. Patients education entails, teaching your patients relevant medical information in a way they understand.

As a nurse, it is your duty to explain medical terminologies to your patients and members of their family. You must be able to explain diseases processes, symptoms, medication, and self-care techniques to your patients and their relatives.

Patient teach-back is a vital patient education technique. Ask patients to repeat a set of instructions or health information in their own words. It will help them assimilate the information and also help you confirm if they truly understand the process.

COMMUNICATION BETWEEN COLLEAGUES OR COWORKERS

It is common to experience occasional conflicts between nurses, especially if there are more stressful periods.

Effective communication in workplaces minimizes misunderstandings and improves work efficiency. People already have personal problems they confront daily at home; don't contribute to the stress they are dealing with. Resolve issues in a collaborative manner.

Here are some tips for fostering healthy communication between nursing colleagues:

1) **Be Culture Sensitive** - Everyone is unique in their own ways. It is common to find a healthcare facility that comprises nurses of various backgrounds, culture, race, religion or ethnicities. Exhibit a professional character; respect each person's uniqueness.

Some people come from countries where individuals speak multiple languages. If your janitor speaks poor grammar or any of your coworkers have a foreign accent, respect the fact that your employers recognized their skills and value to the organization.

2) **Difference in Temperament** – If you work with some individuals long enough, you will discover different reactions to certain situations or reports. Everyone exhibits certain uniqueness that defines who they are.

Some individuals are always lively and quick to forgive any offenses, while others are moody, intolerant, and would prefer their privacy. There are four basic temperaments – sanguine, pragmatics, melancholic, and choleric. Research the differences in these temperaments and know the one you fall in. It will help you understand why people behave the way they do.

3) **Written Communication** - This is important for a nurse. Conveying information to your colleagues in a legible and concise manner explains your level of character and professionalism.

Use approved abbreviations and terminology that is well known. It is also a good way of conveying confidential information.

4) **Active listening** - Show interest in what your colleague has to say. Listen carefully, maintaining eye contact while they speak. It shows you have respect for them.

Texting while your colleague is talking to you could be interpreted as disrespect. When you're in a conversation with another colleague or a group and your phone rings, simply excuse yourself while you leave to answer your call.

Ask questions to clarify issues you may have and always wait for them to finish before you speak.

5) **Apply discretion in your speech** - When you sense a tense atmosphere among coworkers, don't take sides. If you must say something, make sure they are words that will restore calm.

6) **Speak face to face when having a dialogue** - Face to face communication sends the signal of openness and interest in what your colleague has to say. You can read their body language and understand their viewpoint when you speak face to face with them. This also helps to resolve rising conflicts.

7) **Offer constructive criticism** - Be professional in your manner of speaking. Commend a coworker when they do a great job and when they repeat a mistake, offer constructive criticism. Don't make it worse by using a downgrading tone.

8) **Build and earn trust amongst your coworkers** - To establish a healthy relationship among your coworkers, everyone must respect and trust each other. Most groups start with this principle, but the flow is hampered or halted by inconsistency. It's vital that you act consistently and in honesty.

   Communicate clearly with your coworkers. Don't be too quick to act on rumors.

   You are going to be closer to some coworkers than others. Hence you should learn how to keep their personal information confidential. This is a rare quality in people, and it takes discipline not to yield to the temptation to spill. There will be more cooperation and less friction between coworkers when they maintain these professional principles.

9) **Get personal but don't be too casual** - You can get to know your colleagues better, but in the process of gaining closure don't lose your discipline. Ask questions like, "why are you worried?" "Are you okay?" "Is there anything I can do to help?" "What's the good news?" But when you sense withdrawal in their speech, respect their boundaries. You are a nurse after all, and not a spy.

   Avoid the use of offensive language in the workplace. If you are communicating via phone calls or emails, keep it professional.

10) **Consider communication options** - There are various platforms on the internet you can use to maintain communication with your coworkers. You can be consistent in your relationship in and out of the office. However, it all depends on individual preference. Some like using emails, others prefer more social platforms.

11) **Keep your messages via the media direct, short and simple** - Work shifts can sometimes be filled with so many activities that a little distraction can get you off track. If you are calling from home, keep it simple and straight to the point. Don't expect your colleague to listen to

everything that you're trying to tell them. If it's a text, go direct and precise. Your colleague may not have the luxury of time to read through every detail. Avoid giving complicated explanations with the expectation that they will understand or respond immediately.

12) **Maintain Media Etiquette** - Try to be polite via your media or phone calls. If you're unavailable, make sure you've set up a voicemail that is simple and formal. You never know who may call.

When communicating with your colleagues via texts or calls, try to maintain confidentiality. You never know who might be reading.

13) **Appreciate your colleagues when they reach out** - When you're away from work due to personal reasons, appreciate those colleagues who send postcards or texts. A short message in the form of "thanks for reaching out" out of your busy schedule is appropriate.

COMMUNICATING WITH YOUR EMPLOYERS

Healthy communication with your employers also ensures your comfort and effective service delivery. Understand that you're a valuable entity entitled to rights and safe working condition. When those rights are infringed upon, you can sue the organization.

Sometimes, the thought of communicating with your employer(s) is enough to produce stress and anxiety. It takes practice to overcome these fears.

It is beneficial to yourself, and the organization that the communication is between you two is devoid of factors that can debilitate productivity.

The following are tips for effective nurse-employer communication:

1) **Prepare for the conversation** - Before you speak to your employer, write down the lists of items you want to talk about. This will keep your train of thoughts in order and give you the confidence to keep the conversation going.

Engaging personal research boosts your know-how. You will be able to identify problems and offer suggestions that could work. For instance, if your hospital is behind in their software update, you can add that to your discussion with your employer. Offering practical solutions will make you a valuable staff to your management. Also, if you have a meeting with your manager decide whether you would like to implement a new initiative with a group such as hourly rounding or a dermal pressure ulcer reduction protocol. Having new ideas shows that you are committed to improving the unit.

2) **Think through your topics** - Ensure you're clear about the topics you want to discuss with your boss. Time is of the essence, and you do not want to come across as uninteresting or time-wasting.

   Rehearse what you want to say. If you can anticipate the needs of your boss before they arise, you will be seen as a leader and a problem solver. Carry out your research; find out about their upcoming schedules and deadlines, and offer help.

3) **Use the right pronouns and qualifying words** - Make "I" statements instead of "you." For instance, "I need guidance on how to use the new ePCR."

   Also make use of qualifying words such as "maybe," "possibly," "perhaps," etc. Avoid coming out in strong tone by using absolute words like "never," "always," "every" etc. in most of your sentences.

4) **Sort out your emotional problems yourself** - Deal with your emotions before going to your employer. When your emotion is tensed, take some time to cool-off and regain composure. Do not go into a meeting crying or upset. Your boss is most likely not going to be a comforting shoulder to cry on. If you have an issue that is bothering you try to present it without the emotional outbursts. You can your boss have a business relationship so keep it at that level.

5) **Be an active listener** - Learn how to listen and understand what your employer(s) says. Don't be quick to respond. When you're not clear about a point, give your boss some time to end a statement before asking your questions. Also take notes and write down what feedback you are given. Matter of fact create a folder that you can keep all of your meeting notes. This might come in handy if you find yourself in trouble for any reason, having a record of meeting topics will be beneficial.

6) **Keep an open mind** - When having a discussion with your boss, keep an open mind, and be open to compromise. As your employer, you have a lot to learn from their experience in management or other matters.

7) **Practice good body language** - Your non-verbal responses are also essential when communicating with your employers. Maintain eye contact and avoid fidgeting.

8) **Be prompt in your response** - When you're given instructions, be swift to heed them. Same goes for appreciation. When you delay a commendation or appreciation, it loses its value.

9) **Avoid spreading rumors to or about your boss** – Your self-image matters a lot. Don't tarnish your image by spreading rumors to your employer(s). Don't talk behind their back. If it's discovered, it will reduce the trust and respect they had for you.

   Don't complain behind their back. It's an easy way to lose trust. Even though it takes a high level of discipline, resist the urge to talk bad about your employer with your coworkers.

10) **Communicate on a personal level** - It's not necessary that the conversation be health-related. You can discuss ongoing happenings in the news with them when you're on break. Communicating regularly with members of your management makes you feel comfortable and confident around them.

   You can ask personal questions like, "how was your weekend?" or how they are handling a particular situation. It doesn't mean you are friends, it just shows matured you are as a person. People appreciate a genuine interest in issues that concerns them.

Other tips you can engage;

11) Be assertive and not aggressive.
12) Talk to your boss before issues get out of your control.
13) Congratulate your management or employer - when they achieve a notable record or attain any form of good news.

14) **Have a positive attitude.**

15) **Learn how to create a credible presentation with the use of visual aids.**

NURSE - DOCTOR COMMUNICATION

The nurse-doctor relationship is a very crucial subject in healthcare. Conflicts always arise as a result of a misunderstanding between nurses and doctors. Doctors can ask nurses to perform specific tasks, oblivious of the fact that the nurse has multiple tasks that are a priority. This can generate a misunderstanding if there are lapses in their communication.

Fear is a common problem in nurse-doctor communication. As a result of fear, some nurses make medical errors that they could have avoided if they had asked questions.

In some cases, nurses are not to blame when medical errors happen because some doctors have created an air of perfection about them that they dread admitting mistakes. As a result, nurses are cautious not to step on toes.

Nurses are supposed to be the eyes of doctors. Since they are close to the patients, they should be able to spot errors and communicate to the doctors for correction.

TIPS FOR IMPROVING NURSE-DOCTOR COMMUNICATION

The following are suggestions on what you can do to improve communication with the doctors:

1) **Have a sense of value in your profession** - Take pride in your practice by showing up on time, paying attention to details and remain consistent at it. This will make doctors respect you and improve your relationship with them.

   Exercising great levels of professionalism encourages the doctor to be open-minded with you. You need to be proficient in sharing information quickly, reliably, and in a transparent manner. Keep legible notes of your patients and doctors' instructions.

Keeping accurate details will help you retain and disseminate information.

2) **Learn how to organize your information** - Doctors are suckers for organization. They are quickly frustrated when things are not in orderly fashion. Before you relay your information, make sure it is well organized, logical and in a concise manner. Stick to the important details. Doctors are principled when it comes to time management, so leave out the unnecessary details as you communicate the information to them.

3) **Have a positive attitude** - If you want to be respected, exhibit positive behavior. Negative attitudes such as sarcasm, quick-temper, rudeness, etc. are turnoffs. Maintain a positive attitude in order to coexist peacefully.

4) **Be a team player** - Recognize that everyone on your team has a significant role to play. Don't go into any shift with a solitary mentality. Avoid using terms such as "my patient," "your job," etc.

5) **Speak up when you notice any anomaly** - As an aspect of professional character, speak up when you notice an error or a potential error. However, do it in a way that won't escalate the matter.

6) **Assess the context** - Some doctors react to certain situations as a result of accumulated stress Be smart in figuring out when to respond, contribute or ask questions as one statement could tamper with a train of thought. Also, consider the personality of the physician involved and know how to approach the situation.

7) **Have a sense of humor** - There are times that a comic relief can ease tensed situations. This does mean to tell unnecessary jokes in the middle of an operation. A short witty comment after a long period of tensed activity could loosen the stiff atmosphere and create a chance for positive interactions with doctors or surgeons.

8) **Demonstrate some level of friendliness** - Occasionally smile, say hello and ask how doctors are faring. Offer them tea or coffee, and engage them in a brief discussion that might catch their interest.

9) **Set boundaries if you may** - It's okay to be nice and friendly, but also make it clear about certain restrictions. Do this in a respectful way that won't hurt any feelings. Instead of telling a doctor that you don't have time to do what they are asking, say that you will do it after you're done with specific tasks.

   When you have specific observation or insight about a patient, don't be afraid to say it. Your opinion could prove invaluable.

10) **Be precise** - Don't try to impress the doctor with clever medical jargon. Convey information precisely and straight to the point. You do not know the doctor's level of education. Always give them the benefit of the doubt.

DOMINATE HANDOFF REPORT

"A lack of clarity could put the brakes on any journey to success."

Steve Maraboli

Common questions to answer you proceed:

➢ *What is a handoff report?*
➢ *What is the importance of efficient handoff?*

As a nurse, how can I improve the complications associated with handoff reports?

Perhaps one of the toughest tasks you had to do as a new graduate nurse is to provide a good report to the oncoming nurse or charge nurse in the next shift. You know how vital providing accurate relevant information can be for the continuous care and safety of patients.

Caring for patients requires various procedures and as a result, many hands go into their care and recovery. Depending on the nature of the illness or health condition, patients are transferred from one department to another.

To better understand it, think of it this way. Patient "X" is diagnosed by three different specialists. During this diagnosis, a lot of clinical observation, assessment, and tests are reported and communicated between these specialists before the next procedure.

Patient "X" is admitted by the Emergency room who cared for him for several hours.

Patient "X" is then transferred to an Intensive Care Unit where various physicians working could care for him. Remember, these new sets of professionals also need the previous information on Patient "X." Another lapse continues to occur during these routine shifts. Important information is confusing when they are communicated verbally or electronically during the chain of transfers. This can affect the wellness or safety of Patient "X."

Healthcare providers, including nurses, are responsible for care of patients and the continuity of this practice via a process known as handoff. Since there are multiple shifts in an organization, it is vital that nurses get accurate information relevant to their patients at each point of contact.

Inaccurate information could affect work routine and consequently, the care system. The objective of this chapter is to educate on the meaning, importance, and how to prepare a handoff report.

What is a Handoff Report?

As the term suggests, "handoff" simply means to transfer or handover. In a clinical setting, handoff or handoff Report is the transfer of information containing details of all the care processes recorded in a work routine to another transition with the authority and responsibility.

A handoff report is a transfer and acceptance of patient care and responsibility. Patients' specific information is communicated from one caregiver to the other during the transfer of care. This is done to continue the process of patients' safety and care.

The transitioning nurse has the opportunity to ask questions about the previous shifts and any relevant information that will assist them in the new shift.

When this is carefully and efficiently done, there should be a continuous transition process of vital information that results in the continuity of patient care and safety.

Problems Associated with Handoff Reports

The development of the health care system has significantly impacted handoffs. Some generations ago, handoffs were simpler. As a result of the sophistication in today's facility and increased number of physicians, handoffs can be very complicated. As a result of its complex nature, a little lapse can affect patient care and safety.

Most nurses have also identified problems of missing information on handoffs. How do some of these breaches in handoffs happen? It's easy, during report inaccurate medical information is often provided. Such as missing allergies, wrong diagnosis or other pertinent information.

The experience level of a nurse and their interpersonal communication skills also play a significant role in determining a handoff. Since most nursing schools do not teach how to handoff patients, this problem will continue to affect novice nurses until they have a positive learning experience.

This issue has become so disturbing that the Joint Commission introduced a national patient safety goal on handoffs which took effect from January 2006.

Examples of handoff expectations as represented in the guidelines for the implementation of the safety goal by the Joint Commission:

1) A patient who has remained bedridden as a result of a surgical operation since being transferred to the nursing unit. The outgoing nurse reports to the oncoming nurses that the patient will need help getting out of bed, perhaps preventing a patient from falling.

2) Carl (an oncoming nurse on Unit Y) is receiving a report from Linda (another nurse) who is transferring the patient from unit "Y" to unit "Z." The patient MAR (Medication Administration Record) does not show that the patient has received any pain medication in the previous shift. When Carl asks about this, Linda (the outgoing nurse) realizes she gave morphine sulfate but did not enter it in the report or the MAR. As a result of the

question asked by Carl, Linda recognizes the omission and communicates the information and documents it in the MAR. By this action, an overdose of medication has been prevented.

3) Handoff Reports require a process for verification of the received information, and this includes a read back format. Example: the receiver of a telephone message concerning a laboratory value is told to note it down and reread the message starting with the name of the patient, the test, and the test result or interpretation. Details that should be documented should also include the name and credentials of sender and receiver with the time and date.

Lab Technician: "I am calling with the laboratory results on Mr. Felix."

Nurse Linda: "Just a moment, let me get a notepad. Are you calling the lab results for Ms. Anna Whitaker?"

Lab Technician: "No, I am calling the lab results for Mr. Felix Abbeville with ID Number 00267901. Mr. Felix's potassium level is 4.8, drawn at 1900 today.

Nurse Linda: You reported that Mr. Felix Abbeville's potassium level is 4.8. This is Linda Braxton, RN.

Lab Technician: Thank you, Ms. Braxton. That is accurate; Mr. Felix Abbeville's potassium level is 4.8. This is Liam Kendrix, lab technician.

4) A nursing unit plans out staffing coverage to provide for the transition and reduce the potential occurrence of interruptions during the transition report. Assistant nurses do not leave the nursing unit until the report is completed to ensure that phones are answered and prompt response to call lights are made. Nurses provide report successfully as a result.

Suggestions on How to Ensure Quality Handoffs

The best method for giving a timely report is by using a tool such as your patient assignment report form. This document should contain all of the necessary information needed to give a clear description of your client to the on-coming nurse. If you simply read the document from top to bottom it will allow for the receiving nurse to ask follow-up questions and facilitate a healthy dialogue. I will provide an example on the following page.

Here are other tips suggested by experienced clinicians and analysts and how to ensure quality handoffs:

1) Ascertain the crucial information that needs to be communicated

2) Ensure that facility mandated tools are utilized. These come in the form of checklists, templates, protocols, and mnemonics like the I-PASS.

3) Communicate via phone calls or video conference if the direct handoff is not feasible.

4) Ensure that the receiver gets at least these details:
   a. Sender contact information
   b. Allergy list(s)
   c. Code status
   d. Body systems overview
   e. Dated lab tests
   f. Important medications
   g. Details on the vital signs with the date
   h. Nature of illness or illness assessment (including severity)
   i. To-do action list
   j. Contingency plans
   k. Other details such as patient summary (events leading up to illness and admission, hospital course, ongoing assessment)

5) To avoid non-emergency interruptions, conduct your handoff reports as direct as possible.

6) Use technologies like telehealth, applications or patient portals and to make information more readily accessible.

Sample Report Form

RM # 102	RM #
NAME: J. Brown	NAME:
AGE: 55 SEX: M	AGE: SEX:
ISO: TELE: N/A	ISO: TELE:
DX: CHF	DX:
HX: DM II, CA, Smoking	HX:
ALLERGIES: NKDA	ALLERGIES:
CODE STATUS: FULL	CODE STATUS:
ACCU CHECKS: Q 6 HRS	ACCU CHECKS:
DIET: REGULAR	DIET:
MD: Carter	MD:
ACTIVITY: No Restrictions	ACTIVITY:
IV ACCESS: 20 G RUA	IV ACCESS:
NEURO: Alert & Oriented x 4	NEURO:
CARDIO: Normal Sinus Rhythm Last 5:00 PM B/P 150/ 75, HR 80	CARDIO:
RESP: Lungs Clear No Resp Distress	RESP:

GI: Clear Yellow Urine uses urinal	GI:
GU: Abd soft non tender Last BM today 9:00 am	GU:
SKIN: Skin intact Ambulates independently	SKIN:
MISC: Wife visited Last BG was 176 at 6:30 pm	MISC:

DOMINATE YOUR NURSE VALUE

"It's not hard to make decisions when you know what your values are."

Roy Disney

Professional Ethics that Define Who You are as a Nurse

Values can be defined as the characteristics of a subject, person, material, or an idea that makes them desirable. The worth you ascribe to something, that is value.

The general perception can determine value, but values in this context are more individually oriented. Your personal belief, attitude about the quality, perception, and actions you attribute towards a subject is its value. In an auction sale, almost every participant appreciates the item on sale, but only specific individuals are willing to break their banks to acquire it. As valuable as life is, there are still serial killers, suicide bombers and individuals who are ready to end their life if certain things do not go their way. So, you can say, values are actions or sacrifices we input into an idea, thought, person, material, or profession.

As you continue to grow in experience you will inherently increase your value as a nurse professionally. Along with organic work experiences, you must continue to seek out learning opportunities and continuing education.

Once you are on a specific unit for about 2 years you should be able to obtain enough hours of experience to get certified or take a certification test in that area. This will allow you to be a leader on the unit.

Also, take advantage of any degrees or school classes that your hospital/facility may pay for. It is in the best interest of employers to make sure their staff is advancing and able to carry out the latest health practices.

The more knowledge and experience you capture the more marketable you will become as a nurse. After I had 2 years' experience, I was able to take travel nurse assignments where I was paid a premium to work and also got to see many new and exciting places.

Value as a concept of sacrifice

In the face of racial discrimination in the 1800s and early 1900s, Mary Eliza Mahoney amongst others chose to pursue a career in nursing because of her passion for it. Now, not only does history recognize her as the first Registered African American Nurse, but her contributions in the service and her legacies have outlived her.

In the heat of the Crimean war, Mary Seacole persisted in providing care to the injured Jamaican and British soldiers. She was severally rejected to provide care for the British soldiers because of her color, but that didn't stop her. She funded her own course as she continued to provide the medical attention, caregivers, and the best nursing supplies at the time to the wounded during the war.

Beneath the beautiful impression that the nursing profession exudes, there's a lot of complexity that abound in its facets. This explains why some students gave up in the middle of their nursing program. **Unless you match your interest and passion with your actions, value is just an idea.**

You have made it through school and internships, that's awesome. Now is the time to imprint your indelible service into this life-saving career.

Value as a subject

Worth can be measured in numbers. Every item has its varying significance measured by scarcity and monetary price. Value in this sense represents the proportionate worth of an item described in figures.

Determining the value of a thing requires factors such as its peculiarity, scarcity and demand. Some people choose nursing as a career because of its monetary significance. Most parents who influence their children's career prospection often encourage them to go for a highly competitive course like nursing for job security. This is because nurses can work in various organizations, public or private sector.

Morals and nursing practice

Professional scope aside, life will present you with all sort of issues and circumstances that will prompt your reaction. How you confront difficult situations defines your belief system and level of maturity.

In nursing practice, your professionalism is tested on daily basis. You confront challenges in various forms that you've been trained to overcome. From work stress to the difficult tasks and uncooperative patients, it's reasonable to get frustrated at times. It is how you deal with that frustration that depicts who you are and your moral standpoint.

Sometimes, the stress from your personal life could clash with frustrations at the workplace. Being able to survive such times is not easy. This is why its recommended for caregivers to find a support group they can always use as avenue for stress relief. Patients' care and safety require you at your best.

The majority of the challenges you face tests your honesty and ability to make the right decisions.

New graduate nurses often encounter a challenge to their own values and confront circumstances that are new and require them to make decisions that are contrary to their own beliefs. In nursing practice, whether midwifery or clinical practice, healthcare must be filled with discriminatory actions. Issues such as accountability, negligence, and responsibility need to be scrutinized in relation to personal and professional values.

CORE VALUES OF THE NURSING PROFESSION

People dive into the profession for many reasons, but only genuine reasons determine how long you will last in the profession. To say that the profession has its challenges is an understatement.

As a new nurse in practice, understanding these core values helps keep you to have a positive frame of mind and a thorough understanding of your purpose. Knowing who you are defines how you do things.

Nursing is a profession of its own; it is not a subsidiary in the medical practice, that is, it is not inferior to other medical practice. You are a professional caregiver with diverse responsibilities in the field.

Your values are not restricted. What are those fundamental aspects of the profession that defines what you represent? What separates you from other caregivers?

Excellence in caring

One of the core values in the nursing profession is the virtue and dedication to quality care to clients. It is like a culture. Nurses remain committed to constant understanding, growth, and development of care system.

Precise and accurate care is an ethical value in nursing profession. Nurses carry out their tasks in a thoughtful manner, based on competent clinical skills and nursing knowledge to ensure patients' safety.

The longer you continue in the practice, you begin to realize how much you have transformed and your growing distaste for mediocrity.

Critical Thinking

Critical thinking is an active cognitive process engaged in the mind for decision making. Reasoning, meditations, and well-defined thought processes are exercised to achieve results in an appropriate time frame.

Nursing practice can be quite delicate in the toughest of times. Your discernment and mental concentration need to be at maximum level. A little distraction can result in irreparable damage.

As a nurse, you are constantly involved in clinical decision making that requires aptness, promptness, and precision. You must be able to think critically when timely decisions are of the essence.

The unpredictability aspect of the job requires that you stay focused irrespective of the emotional state you were in. Quick decisions may be mandatory in some cases. However, the accuracy of your decision is of utmost importance.

To ensure the outcomes of your decision are error-free, you need to engage your team. Engage a teamwork approach to problem-solving. When a situation is way over your head, don't hesitate to ask questions and make notes of the lessons you receive daily.

Among other things, critical thinking explores essential possibilities without indulging in assumptions. Factors that will aid decision-making process includes past experiences, research endeavors, and knowledge base.

As you continue to gain experience in practice, you will be able to think independently, persist in the face of difficult challenges, trust your instinct, and manage risks effectively.

Selflessness

This is a common trait in nursing from the era of Florence Nightingale. **Nurses have a culture of putting the needs of their patients first**. The trait of consideration for humans as the pivot of attention and focus has survived many generations.

Nurses are natural altruists. Once that connection between clients and nurses are established, the desire to help them through their recovery process takes over.

Caring and Empathy

Another core value in the nursing profession is the ability to empathize and show compassionate care. This quality emanates from a deep understanding. It is a fundamental aspect of nursing practice.

Even when it is not apparent facially, nurses care deeply about their patients. It is this sensitivity to the patients' condition that provokes the willingness and zeal to help patients recover from their illness. Nurses can manage their emotions because they understand the importance of staying focus.

It is this empathy and compassion that improves communication between nurses and patients.

When you take interest in the growth, well-being, and recovery of your patients, empathy will come naturally. It begins to show in your body language, actions, and expressions of hope.

As a fundamental aspect of nursing profession, caring comes top of the list. Nurses show concern and consideration for everyone no matter their belief, language, or background.

The whole organization's activity is people-centered; demonstrating commitment to understand and care for the needs of the people.

Teaching

Another value in the nursing practice is teaching. Nurses educate their patients and their families the meaning of some medical terminologies. Most times, doctors speak in a language that may be difficult for a patient to understand, this will require a nurse to break it down to their level.

Nurses also teach patients and families how to use certain drugs, the effects, and precautionary measures. Nurses assess their needs and provide them with accurate information that is relevant to their care. Whether you are a registered nurse or practical nurse be prepared to teach.

Diversity

The nursing profession is all-embracing, promoting excellence in diverse ethnicity, race, gender, socio-economic status, physical abilities, religion, age, etc. the professional ethic also addresses behaviors in the health and academic sectors.

No one calls for "the Latin American girl," or "the tall African American" in a hospital. Everyone is either addressed as Nurse or by their names. Differences affect development negatively, so such unprofessional trait is never encouraged in this 21st century.

Therapeutics

This involves the treatment of disabilities or disease, mentally or physically. Nurses apply medically approved therapeutic procedures to cases where related. These applications can be nutritional or pharmacological. This is based on the knowledge of the uses of such therapy and skills in patient evaluation.

Nurses use nutritional modality in therapy when it is medically prescribed.

Trust

Ability to believe, confide, and rely on the treatments of professional nurses comes naturally because nurses possess an appealing virtue that inspires hope. It's a nursing ethical value since nursing exhibit traits of honesty in words and practice.

Nurses establish trust by understanding a patient's situation and health status. It is not just the patients, the families, and the society also trusts the nursing practice.

Integrity

Professional nurses demonstrate character and dignity. Healthcare organization are established on principles and integrity.

Trust work both ways, you can't entrust your family member or yourself into the wrong hands when you need medical treatment. Nurses consistently demonstrate moral integrity and professional standards in their practice.

Psychomotor Skills

Nurses, through the knowledge they have acquired in nursing school, can assess mental impulses and evaluate patients' health status (by using their hands) to provide comfort to patients. This skill is used in a manner that boosts the comfort of the patients.

Psychomotor skills provide the highest level of accuracy of information and an effective result on the health status of the patients. It gets better through practice.

Autonomy in decision making

Registered nurses exercise autonomy in decision making by providing adequate information to patients and also suggest diagnosis and treatments. The right to accept or reject suggested treatment procedures is reserved for experienced nurses.

Nurses explain suggested nursing interventions and give patients the options to accept or reject procedures. Sometimes, families also participate in this decision-making process.

Responsibility

Commitment to patients' care and safety on a daily basis is ethical virtue in nursing profession. Nurses are responsible for providing the best clinical function, evidence-based-care through clinical research, and show accountability for their actions and duties.

Promoting patients' well-being via a comprehensive approach is a responsibility in nursing practice.

Human relationship

Sympathy, sincerity in words, politeness, and mutual understanding ensure effective nurse-patient relationships.

From the moment a patient gets admitted into the hospital, gets treated and discharged after successful treatment, there's a steady communication between nurses and the patients. Nurses demonstrate traits of trust and mutual respect for everyone.

As an ethic in practice, nurses uphold patients' confidentiality and privacy agreement. This practice guarantees trust in the nurse-patient relationship.

Legal tenets

There is a professional standard guiding the nursing practice. The standards are well defined by the statutory, regulatory, and common law.

Nurses abide by their ethics. Health care services such as medication, treatment, and patient assessment by a nurse are within the professional ethics and legal boundary. Nurses go around with this principle like a uniform.

It is common knowledge that professional nurses exhibit qualities such as responsibility, patience, justice, confidentiality, kindness, sincerity, fidelity, and accountability. By showing these traits, it enhances their ability to practice ethically.

106

As a nurse, you must understand the legal boundaries that protect your client and your own right. Otherwise, you might be sued for unprofessional conducts such as battery, negligence, malpractice, etc.

Individual and professional competency

This is an ethical value in the nursing profession that calls for professional competence so that nurses can acquire the necessary skills and certifications. Nurses go for individual training to grow and develop their knowledge base and proficiency in the use of new technologies.

The profession promotes personal competency and development in order to acquire up-to-date knowledge, practical skills, use of clinical skills, and the ability to provide comprehensive care. There are various continuous programs in multiple countries that nurses participate in, nursing rankings include nursing assistant, CAN, Licensed Professional Nurse (LPN), RN, Advanced Practice Registered Nurse (APRN), Doctor of Nursing Practice (DPN) in that order.

Health is a serious business, and the nursing body takes it very seriously. Healthcare organizations also promote personal and professional expertise when nurses prove resourceful or indicate interest. Participation in continuing professional advancement to preserve competence and efficiency in health care is encouraged.

DOMINATING YOUR CAREER AND PERSONAL LIFE
(Balancing Personal Life with Professional life)

"Consider it pure joy, my brothers and sisters, whenever you face trials of many kinds, because you know that the testing of your faith produces perseverance. Let perseverance finish its work so that you may be mature and complete, not lacking anything."

James 1:2-4

The Silent Killer at Your Workplace

A lot has been discussed about the stress nurses face at workplaces, especially new graduate nurses. Stating the emphasis on how this can affect productivity in the organization is apparently not enough.

The organization you work for will outlive your existence. You are replaceable, whether you work through retirement age or exit via resignation. As soon as you walk out the door, someone is contacted to take your spot. This is why you should pay close attention to your health.

Your health is very important to the organization, your clients, your loved ones, and yourself. It will be unwise on your part to ignore these facts with the excuse that you are too busy.

Work-related stress can be subtle. Sometimes you may not realize it until the signs begin to surface. It lurks in the shadows, draining your energy, distorting your concentration, and diminishing your confidence. You get so absorbed with your tasks and intent to impress your superior officials that you don't notice the early symptoms. Your colleagues notice and talk about it in hushed tones. The ones who care at all inform you, but you are not convinced.

What is Stress?

Stress is the accumulation of emotional or physical pressure on the body. Stress can be psychological too.

Studies have shown that excess stress can lead to physical symptoms such as headaches, high blood pressure, pain in the chest, insomnia, stomach upset. Stress can also cause mood disorders like anxiety and depression.

Stress is in two forms – the good and bad stress. Also called "eustress," the good stress is vital for boosting productivity in the workplace. It acts as an added push or motivation in workers. Bad stress or distress, on the other hand, limits individual outputs. Distress is exhausting and occurs when the good stress builds up and becomes excessive.

Factors that contribute to stress at workplaces

1) Pressure due to nature of task. When a task is too complex, and there's little or no guidance, it can stress you mentally.

2) Pressure to impress your superior officials or management

3) Fear of being laid off or fired.

4) Accumulated stress from working overtime.

5) Pressure to continually work at peak levels. This can come from personal set goals or intention to impress someone

6) Pressure from constantly rising expectations

How to Identify Stress When It Gets Out of Control

The following are warning signs indicating that you need medical attention:

1) **Trouble focusing** - symptoms such as forgetfulness will begin to occur making one lose concentration from time to time. When you notice this symptom, get help immediately as it could have an adverse result on your care process and the patients' safety.

2) **Depressed Mood** - Some individuals mildly refer to it as mood swings at the onset. But it's safer to deal with it at the early stage. Signs such as becoming irritable, experiencing withdrawal, losing confidence, and being in the state of paranoia can affect your performance negatively if you don't deal with them on time.

3) **Possessing a sense of apathy** - Losing interest at something you usually had passion for, your enthusiasm and passion just begin to diminish all of a sudden.

4) **Insomnia** - This is a symptom of unrest; it's a disorder that indicates sleep deprivation. It also has an adverse effect on work performance. You're unable to sleep or experience fatigue during the day

5) **Physical strains** - headaches, muscle tension, stomach problems, etc.

6) **Sexual performance** - when you begin to notice a decrease in your libido, it could be a sign of stress.

Stress Relieving Mechanisms

There are some effective ways of managing stress. Don't resort to food, drugs or alcohol as a coping mechanism. Instead of relieving your stress, it's only making it worse. Here are a few methods for learning how to relieve stress:

1) **Engage in regular exercise** - Isn't it ironic to suggest physical activity as a way of dealing with accumulated pressure? But this method has been proven to be effective in combating stress. With its mood-boosting and endorphin-releasing properties, habitual aerobic exercise is a natural stress reliever.

Regular exercise helps to lighten the mood. Just like antidepressants, exercise reduces the likelihood of feeling depressed.

It gets your mind off your stressful thoughts. Special exercise patterns like the one done at aerobic classes helps to keep you focused, rather than mulling over your worries most of the time. Your mind is engaged in activity resulting in a state of calm mentally and physically.

Make a habit of exercising yourself for a minimum of 30 minutes daily.

It's common for nurses to on their feed for their entire shift. Try to break up this time by alternating sitting and standing if possible.

2) **Engage in positive relationships** - Most therapy sessions set up for stress relief engages individuals to speak up. Stress can be alleviated by merely talking about it. The therapist starts by asking specific questions that relate to the root causes of the problem. You will realize at the end of the session, you've succeeded in releasing the negative vibes off your system.

This is why it's crucial that you only have positive relationships. They might not solve your problems, but they create avenues for you to talk your stress away. The simple act of confiding in someone you can trust and verbalizing your fears, worries, anxieties, and pressure can actually reduce the severity.

Also, good friends can take your mind off your source of worry. Having healthy interactions, humor, and positive conversations engage your mind and keep it from harmful thoughts.

3) **Eat healthy and Nutritious Foods** - When we are stressed, the brain releases the hormone cortisol. This hormone makes us crave sweet, salty, and fatty foods like pizza, ice cream, burgers, cheese, red meat, etc. This is not safe for our health. Such kind of food causes the body to be sluggish.

Eat whole foods because processed foods can cause us to feel anxious and can even contribute to weight gain. By eating whole foods, more fruits and vegetables help to prevent symptoms of work stress.

Also, getting a healthy dose of omega-3 fatty acids from salmon or seeds such as hemp and flax will help to prevent symptoms. Nourishing your body will prepare you to overcome the challenges you will encounter at your work routine.

Avoid taking caffeinated drinks because it impedes your ability to sleep. Also avoid nicotine substances, alcohol, and other depressants.

The safe thing to do is to eat complex carbohydrate (like whole-wheat bread, vegetables or pasta) that boosts our brains. This will help us concentrate and learn how to overcome work-related stress.

Other examples of food you can eat include:
- lean proteins like chicken,
- high fiber foods such as vegetables and fruits,
- blueberries, dark chocolates, kale, etc.

4) **Learn the habit of saying "No" and standing by it** - Recognize that humility is not the same as foolishness. **Humility is doing what is right at the right time.** If you allow yourself to get overbooked, overworked, and overcommitted just to please everyone, you will be stressed out.

It's common to feel obligated to honor your word. But the greatest act of stress relief is exercising your right to say no. You can be polite but be firm. Explain why you can't do certain things. You can say, "I'm sorry ma'am, my shift is done. Nurse Tiffany is taking over from here."

Briefly explain to them that you can't do it because you are overcommitted at the moment. Don't leave your boss out of this equation, you can say "no" to your boss. Just explain that one more project will result in a drop in the quality of your work.

5) **Get Enough Sleep** - Poor sleep contributes to stress. You should try getting at least 6 hours of sleep in every 24 hours. Inadequate sleep causes poor concentration and consequently, poses a risk in your care process.

When you deprive your body of sleep, it causes irritability and the risk of being unable to combat stress.

Having enough rest will keep your mind refreshed and able to perform at peak. One common trait with most creative people is that they get adequate rest, enabling them to have full concentration. The fact that a simple error could cost the safety of a patient is enough reason to give your body the adequate rest it requires, keeping the mind at its best.

6) Don't Lose Sight of Your Purpose - Our purpose is bigger than the work we do. Everyone has a distinctive purpose, whether as a midwife or med-surgical nurse. We are creative, in relationships, spiritual, and passionate in various ways. Connecting with our whole selves by maximizing our sense of purpose is the basis for less stress and more happiness, professionally and otherwise.

What does this mean? How does purpose relate to stress or stress relief? Purpose simply means vision. Can you imagine how stressful life will be without your sight? Without someone aiding you from post to post? That's how stressful a purposeless life is. Purpose can be described as a person's calling on earth. But it is actually broader than that.

Purpose comprises of everything from meaningful work to relationships, to less important things such as the little things we do and derive joy and meaning from.

Purpose is the manifestation of our own unique spirit. When we fail to follow this ordained path by not engaging with our work, suppressing our creativity or disregarding our relationships, we automatically set off a life of stress and struggle.
If you take away the relationships and the creative potentials, all that will be left is a life of obligations. Such lifestyle is laden with struggles, bitterness, resentment, depression, and paranoia.
The solution to these negativities is to discover your purpose and focus on it. You will not just live with a stress-free life, but a meaningful one too.

What to do:

a) Set out your quality social time: so often, nurses get so preoccupied with their crazy work routine, sacrificing the time for their relationship or personal life. Learn how to apportion some time for your relationship or personal life (This will be discussed further).

b) Be creative. Growing up, we exhibited innovative attributes. There is a certain level of creative intelligence in everyone. As we grow, some of us continue to improve through practice or relinquish it for other interests.
But it's essential to make out time to hone this creative ability just for leisure. This can include anything from cooking dinner, painting, sending a special card to a friend, or creating a vision board. Get out your scissors and glue stick and just have fun.

c) Get spiritual. Irrespective of what the term "spirituality" means to you. One thing is for sure: When you are overworked and continually stressed, you can forget about your place in the bigger picture.

A great way of comprehensively grasping and relieving your stress is by connecting with your spiritual roots. You can do this through prayer, chanting or meditation.

The following are tactics that you can use

-   Set out your goals: before prioritizing your tasks, clarify your objectives. You can get the help of a more experienced nurse who has been in the facility before you. As you work, reevaluate your shift to know if you reached your set goal.

-   Focus on a maximum of 2 goals at a time: When you have identified the two things that are of utmost important, focus on them. This will improve your self-confidence when you have reached those set goals. Setting your mind on more than 3 goals will distort your concentration and contribute to stress.

- Set a realistic deadline: This will help you manage your time and avoid encroaching into the timeline of the on-coming nurses. Setting a realistic deadline does not just ensure your task and goals are accomplished, but the feeling that comes with completing a task is stress relieving

- Make a To-Do List: Write down the list of things you plan to get done. This sort of arrangement fixes the problem of forgetfulness and loss of concentration.

- Even if your to-do list extends up to 50 tasks, you need to prioritize those tasks into four categories.

   They are:
   - Urgent and important
   - Important but not urgent
   - Urgent but not important
   - Neither urgent nor important.

Know your chronotype

If you are a morning person, though, high-concentration tasks should be your top priority in the morning. Don't attend to tough tasks during night time and vice versa.

- Use your calendar: Plan your weeks within your calendar to optimize the use of time. Also, schedule your breaks in there.

How to balance Professional and Personal life

As exhausting as mental stress can be, it is manageable. As a new nurse, learning how to handle work-related stress and keeping your personal life from interfering with our professional life can be tough. It even gets worse if you have multiple commitments. For example, if you are a single mother of 2 kids with a new man in your life, it will take a while getting used to the new job.

This problem is not often addressed. The nursing school is more concerned about teaching you the basics in your nursing practice. The responsibility of stress management falls largely on you.

Other reasons why this problem is still at large in most healthcare organizations is because most individuals fail to address the dangers it can cause. Individual's low sense of achievement, lack of career management and cynicisms inhibits on their performances. When these problems are dealt with appropriately, nurses will give their highest level of care for their patients, and it will translate to longevity and happiness for these medical professionals.

Unfortunately, burnout has affected work efficiency, productivity, marriages, relationships, and causes of depression have been on the increase. Some have even quit the practice as a result of its severity.

Mental and physical fatigue has impacted nursing professionals immensely. One of the usual problems is compassion fatigue. This is when nurses feel ill or distressed emotionally. Emotional connections with patients suffering various natures of medical conditions ranging from acute to terminal cases can result in distress and fatigue on the caregivers over time.

The status of your personal life also affects your work performance. If you have a healthy relationship, in good terms with your spouse or kids, it will reflect well on your output. There are few tips on how to establish and maintain a healthy personal and professional life –

1) **Take a break from your work** - The most important factor in a relationship (either with spouse, kids or friends) is time. Relationships begin to experience frictions when there's limited time allotted to it. It takes time to bond and establish other features like trust, love, and friendship. **When you try to explain away your lack of time, you often get "don't worry, I understand" but don't be deceived by that.** There is a little truth in the popular saying that "absence makes the

heart grow fonder." That works when you are away for a while. A long stretch of your absence gradually erases the bond you have established. This explains why some kids are closer to hired babysitters than their biological parents. They are the reason why you are out there working overtime, trying to secure a better future for them. But don't lose them in the process.

At a time when productivity at the workplace is heavily prioritized, taking a break may seem like a leisurely indulgence. As a nurse, the nature of your job comes with increasing activities and piles of paperwork at your desk. Taking a break will enhance your creativity and optimize your focus. Taking a break to have time for your personal engagements will also make you more efficient when you return to work.

If you keep waiting for the perfect time, it may never come. There's no consensus on how regularly nurses should take periodic breaks. However, getting that break when you do will give you adequate time to rest, reinvigorate, and return back, feeling more in control.

2) **Find a Support Group** - Support groups have proven invaluable in the lives of professionals. Whatever reason you go there for, whether to sort out personal problems o work-related issues, you don't return the same. Nurses improve their performances when they participate in social support structures. The benefit translates to increased productivity within the organization. Support groups also abide by confidential agreement which makes members free to express themselves. Speaking about your problem is the first positive step in dealing with it and countering the effects of burnout.

3) **Dedicate Time to Yourself** - Efficiency in your job requires you at your best. Even robots are serviced from time to time. Working long hours at a stretch could cause a breakdown. It is recommended that you dedicate some time to rejuvenate your system.
Learn how to separate personal time from work time. Let your roommates or family members understand how crucial it is for you. If you don't watch it, your work and other issues will just keep encroaching into your personal time. Keep your phones and other gadgets away during these periods.

4) **Keep track of time** - At the initial stage of your transition into practice, you were nervous and uncertain about your future to some extent. But you learned a lot in the space of time and regained confidence. Your interest grows daily, and every day you wake up, your first thought is about your patients. And as you dominate every challenge that comes along, you get engrossed into your work. The next thing you should dominate is how to keep track of time.

Learn to monitor the time you spend on a particular task. Keeping track of time is a good time management strategy that ensures efficiency and productivity. Distractions can come from various angles. You can be on a particular assignment when an emergency case comes to you. Also, keep your phone away when you're on duty.

Providing quality patients' care requires that you improve your time management techniques. Dedicating time to yourself at intervals, does not reduce your productivity.

BUDGETING: PLANNING YOUR FINANCES AS A NEW NURSE

A bad financial plan also contributes to stress and struggles. Dominating your nursing career will require more than learning interesting skills for nursing practice. You are bound to have responsibilities and commitments that will take a tangible share in your consciousness. You need to be in your best (mentally or otherwise) to ensure quality healthcare delivery. Learn how to make proper budgeting so that you can have a good sleep no matter how limited the time.

Learning to budget is very essential as you adjust to full-time practice. A good budget plan guarantees less stress. There's a big difference between your current budget plan and the one you were familiar with in school. Back in college, you probably learned how to allocate money for loan payments and other expenses. Your current status comprises of a lot more responsibilities. Now, you're required to be a bit more organized. More money, more budgeting.

The following are tips to ensure you keep a good budgeting scheme as you transition to full-time nursing practice

1) **Understand the Benefits Your Organization Offers** - When you accepted your job offer, the next thing you did was to discuss the salary and benefits before giving your signature of acceptance. Understanding the details of your contract is very vital. If you're still not sure of how it works, you can contact the Human Resource Manager to go over them again.

A proper understanding of your financial entitlements allows you to take advantage of your benefits. This can reduce your taxable income allocate extra savings. Make a habit of reviewing your benefits each year.

2) **Calculate and track your Expenses** - One characteristic popular among new employees is the inability to account for expenses they make monthly. Ignoring your spending will keep you wondering where all the money went once you're done. Keeping track of your expenses enables you to strategize your budget.

   There are various means you can get it done – either by documenting them using a note or creating a database with special apps on your device. The objective is to ascertain how much you spend over a period of time and compare them with your monthly income.
   Without proper documentation, it's easy to live under false assumptions. When this is the case, it could affect how you think and behave, consequently reflecting on your performance at work.

   The first thing to do is to list out your sources of income unless you have a single income. If you have additional income from private practice or other sources, add them to your list. Next, add up your monthly expenses, such as your utility bills, rent, loan payments, charity, grocery expenses, etc. If there are additional expenses like social outings, going to the movies, booking dinner reservations, etc. add them to the list too.

   The next thing to do is subtract your expenses from your total income. If there's any money left, it should go to the savings column. But if you realize that the remainder is in the negative or there's nothing left, there's your lesson to minimize expenses next time.

   To be even more proactive set up an automatic withdrawal from your account that will go right into a saving account and then live off the remainder. I would have 175 dollars taken out of every paycheck to go into savings. I didn't really miss the money and was able to save up pretty quickly.

3) **Keep Your Monthly Costs Low** - The probability of having more bills and responsibilities is certain as you adjust to the real world. Bills like rent, loan payments, car payments, health insurance, internet subscriptions, utility bills, etc. are good example. Among the list highlighted, your rent is the largest monthly cost. Endeavor to keep that cost as low as you can.

There's always an urge to spend more or improve on your living standard. Try not to live above your means. If your rent is way above your means, you can consider getting a roommate. Depending on your income, you can choose to a more conducive choice that suits your taste. But whatever you do, resist the temptation to start big or above your income.

4) **Be Selective About Your Monthly Subscriptions** - We live in the 21st centuries and so are privileged to have access to multiple fun packages and media utilities. There are varieties of monthly subscription packages to choose from – Netflix, Hulu, HBO, Spotify, etc. Study the packages for their programs and prices. Remember to stick to a plan that won't affect your budget adversely. You can cut down on your subscription packages to minimize expenses and save money.

5) **Watch Against Window Shopping** - Always stick to your budget plan. Resist the temptation to get items every now and then. If this has become a habit that is proving too difficult to curtail, you can hide your credit card in your home before leaving for work.

You can consult a banker to help you set up a fixed deposit account to ensure you have savings at the end of the month.

6) **Be Careful with Compulsive Spending** - Be careful about how you plan some fun activities, like going to watch games, traveling, music shows, shopping, etc. Check to ensure that your budget is not affected.

These activities and other recreational programs might be a good way to relieve stress, but living above your budget could worsen rather than alleviate your stress. The habit you inculcate now will determine how you live in the long run.

7) **Set Up a Savings Plan** - Allocate at least 15 percent of your total income for your savings account. A savings account is a great place to keep cash that you don't plan to spend immediately. These types of accounts keep your money safe and accessible and accrue interests per time, but there are varieties of savings accounts to choose from. Each variation (and bank or credit union) has different features, so it's essential to understand your options.

Study the following account types to find the one that suits you!

a. **Savings Deposits:** this is the most popular type of account. The conditions are simple and easy to understand. They are interest-bearing accounts that allow you to withdraw money at any time. Depending on the type of bank, you have limited transfers per month. This includes transfers to third parties or to other account accounts

b. **Jumbo Savings account:** Similar to Savings account except for the difference in the size of deposits allowed. Deposits permitted in this account are from $100,000 and above. The interest rate for Jumbo Savings is high.

c. **High-Interest Savings Accounts:** As the name suggests, the interests paid to this account are relatively high. There are requirements that secures these interests – high minimum balance or limited withdrawals per month, etc.

d. **Joint Savings Account:** this is a savings account that is jointly held by two or more individuals. There are certain benefits attached to this type of account.

e. **Rewards Savings account:** thins kind of account offers special incentives under certain conditions. Some of which includes reaching a specific level balance, account opening package, etc. it is recommended that you always calculate the value of rewards as a percentage of your balance and include them in any interest rate comparison when opening your savings account.

f. **Student Savings Account:** as the name suggests, banks offer these kinds of accounts to students in high school or universities. Student Savings have more flexible features, terms, and conditions. It also offers low minimum balance requirements.

g. **Certificates of Deposits:** Not a very popular account. This type of account requires you to entrust your savings for a specified time, which may be from one month to several years depending on your agreement.

The maximum number of years in most cases is 5years. You earn higher rates in Certificate of Deposits account package compared to a savings account. It's also a good saving option because your money is not made available to you anytime you want it, unlike the Savings Account, withdrawing before the specified period attracts a penalty.

h. **College Savings Account:** This type of account is set up to aid undergraduates with tuition fees and other expenses.
Another advantage that comes with this type of account is that it is allowed to grow tax-free. As long as they are used for educational purpose, they are not taxed deductible.

i. **Individual Retirement Plan:** this account package allows individuals to withdraw up to five thousand to six thousand, five hundred dollars ($5000 - $6,500) per year.

Upon withdrawal, the account owner is subject to ordinary income tax. When you withdraw before the specified age of retirement, you are penalized in addition to the income tax.

j. **Roth IRA:** This account plan is similar to the same contribution limits as the traditional IRAs. One of the benefits is that contributions are not tax-deductible. You get the benefit on the backend of allotments not being subject to income tax.

k. **401(k) retirement plans:** This plan is sponsored by employers. It allows you to remit up to eighteen thousand dollars ($18,000) of your income before tax for retirement savings.
These plans often feature an employer match of some of your contribution to your 401(k)-retirement savings plan. Your earnings can grow as tax-free savings. Allotments from these plans are subject to income tax. Withdrawals made before the specified retirement age is penalized.

l. **Health Savings Accounts (HSAs):** Almost like an insurance plan, this package allows the account owner to make tax-deductible contributions. You also grow your savings tax-free and pay zero tax on withdrawals as long as they are specified for medical expenses. Participation in this plan subject to your enrollment in a high-deductible health plan.

You are recommended to review this plan with your banker to understand all its features. You will most likely find yourself using a few of these savings accounts at the same time, each designed for a specific purpose.
The important thing is, there are multiple ways to find the most preferable saving account choice if you are looking for ways to save money.

8) **Save 15% of your income** - As a new graduate nurse, understand the importance of setting apart income for your saving account.
Starting and maintaining this habit consistently secures your financial future. In addition to that, having a reliable saving plan puts your mind at ease.

FREQUENTLY ASKED QUESTIONS

- **WHY ARE THERE FEWER MEN IN THE NURSE PROFESSION?**

It is a misguided perception to that the nursing profession is biased. However, it is not a hidden fact to admit that there are more women in the profession. Nursing is more of a caregiver mentality – a trait that is less dominant in men.

The following are some reasons put together by some clinical experts:

1) **Men are more physical than flexible** - Men are more physical and tend to pursue a career that favors such feature. The nursing profession is, however, less adrenaline and much more constant pouring out of oneself to meet physical, spiritual, and emotional needs of others. As a result, it is less appealing to men except in the Emergency Room or trauma units.

2) **Nursing practice has no place for one task mentality** - Women are known to have the ability to multitask. Unlike women, men are task-oriented, usually one task at a time. The nursing practice is quite complicated and rarely has the "one task at a time" mentality.

3) **Widely Accepted concept** - The idea that women are natural caregivers has become so rooted in families that it is difficult to change that mentality. Change of culture requires time and due respect for those who put themselves second. Many see it as a weakness.

- **HOW CAN I GET EXTRA INCOME AS A NURSE?**

The nursing profession provides more than 3 million RNs in the United States alone, with a variety of workplace choices and impressive remunerations.

According to a BLS report in 2016, an average nursing salary for registered nurses ranges from $65,000 - $70,000 per year. Also, the job growth rate between 2014 and 2024 is expected to rise by 16%, which is higher than the average for most professions.

Although financial factor is not the main driving force for most nurses who enter the profession, there are so many options for registered nurses who want to know ways of making extra incomes.

Options are available for nurses to choose from, whether immediate or short term. This includes taking nursing side jobs or becoming a temporary travel nurse.

Basic Ways Nurses make money:

1) **Complete your BSN degree** - A lot of opportunities are available for RNs. Most organizations are on the lookout for positions such as Registered nurses or Entry Level Nurses BSN degrees.

2) **Experienced nurses in a nursing specialty** - Specialty nurses are also on high demand by big healthcare organizations. You should decide on a nursing specialty that will meet your professional and personal goals. You can then proceed to complete certification courses, thereby increasing your knowledge and skills. It has been proven that certified nurses have a better chance to earn higher salaries in their fields.

   Some nurse specialties also offer great remuneration packages compared to others. You can do your research early in your career to identify the right path to choose.

3) **Volunteer to work overtime on occasion** - Engaging in some overtime duties not only provides more money-making opportunities but can prove to your management that you're a team member who'll pitch in when needed. Have it mind that too much overtime can lead to stress; however, you can set out reasonable limits to monitor yourself and your patients.

4) **Get an advanced nursing degree** - Getting an advanced nursing degree will give you an edge over other competitions. You can earn solid income practicing as an advanced practice registered nurse (APRN), nurse manager, or other professional.

APRNs require a master's degree (MSN), and you can further your practice independently. Good examples are the clinical nursing specialists (CNS), nurse practitioners (NP), certified registered nurse anesthetist (CRNA), certified nurse midwife (CNM). According to the U.S Bureau of Labor Statistics, the CRNAs make the highest average salaries among all APRNs, averaging close to $160,000.

Other career opportunities with a master's or doctoral degrees involve working as a nurse educator or finding your way up the ranks in health care administration.

5) **Get creative with nursing side jobs** - There is a variety of savvy jobs you can engage for extra incomes. If you are deciding to earn income through nursing side jobs, here is a list of them:

- Proving care for homebound patients

- Working per time shifts on any of your off days.

- Teaching patients how to use medical equipment at home

- You can work as a camp nurse during your vacation days

- Writing blogs

- Giving vaccinations at doctor's offices or specialized clinics

- Teaching patient education classes

6) **Become a travel nurse** - Most experienced nurses can earn income by getting hired by touring groups like musical crews, sports teams, agencies, etc. for their events. Specialty nurses can receive excellent compensation as a travel nurse. Travelers work temporary contracts in various locations around the world.

If one of your top priorities include making more money as a nurse, ask your nursing recruiter to link you up with the best paying assignment, or do a personal research online.

Earning money by becoming a nurse tutor

This is another legitimate way of making a good side income. The location also plays a considerable role. If you live close to a local college that offers any kind of nursing degrees, you can consider offering your services as a tutor. It's a reliable side hustle that also affords you chance to meet people in your field and learn more while teaching. You'll earn a substantial sum and also help someone who is going through a similar situation you had in the past.

You can charge a certain fee per semester or on an hourly basis, which is totally up to you. You don't have to wait till when the opportunity comes. Talk to your former colleagues in Nursing school, professors, and hose in your management team about your interest to teach.

You can earn a side income by becoming a health coach

This is a fun way to make extra money. It involves working directly with clients and helping them improve their health. For example, there are several army veterans that require the services of a health coach.

You can charge on an hourly basis.

Earning side income as a legal nurse consultant

Team up with a lawyer you know or check into a law firm and offer you expertise as a consultant on any health-related case they might be working on.

As a legal nurse consultant, you can share health care knowledge with lawyers get paid per case that you help with. The following are examples of cases you can assist with:

- Personal injury
- malpractice suits
- insurance fraud

You can also earn side income as a substitute school teacher

This is an opportunity for nurses that like working with kids. Talk to some school managers about your interest and leave your business card with them.

You can also check with your local, or state for minimum requirements. The minimum requirement is often a Bachelor's degree.

You can earn income working per-time at retail outlets

This could be fun for you too. Depending on the season, retail shops are usually less crowded with activities. It is not as busy as in a hospital. You can also be paid hourly or weekly wages.

Earning Income as a Travel Agent

You can put your organizational skills to good use working as a travel agent. Another advantage is that you need to operate. Simply get a laptop and get all the information you need to start up the business. Travel agents get paid commissions on the sales made.

Earn extra income working as a home health educator

As a home health educator, you can earn a side income by just teaching basic health information. Charge people for helping them know what you do for a living (patient education).

Earn Extra Income working as a Camp Nurse

This is a popular side job for nurses. Working as a camp nurse also affords you time to relax and have fun doing what you enjoy. The most popular time for camps is obviously the summer. Get paid on hourly basis working as a camp nurse in one of your vacations.

You may need to plan your schedule weeks before the due date.

Other opportunities include:

- Dog walking
- Selling Art
- Virtual assistant
- Babysitting

- **WHAT IS THE DIFFERENCE BETWEEN LPN AND RN?**

Most LPNs feel inferior when they are transitioning into full-time practice. It's important to know that each rank is as important as the responsibilities. Medical duties are expertly carried out as a team. The efforts of each individual, whether LPN, RN, or APRN is invaluable towards ensuring the safety and wellbeing of patients. It's, however essential to understand the difference in other not to displace the value and the roles that each one plays.

The acronym 'LPN' represents - "Licensed Practical Nurse." LPN is the most basic kind of nurse. In some states in the USA (specifically, California and Texas), an LPN is referred to as "LVN," meaning *Licensed Vocational Nurse*.

A major difference between Licensed Practical Nurses and Registered Nurses is that the LPN requires a less formal program. An LPN may not be given responsibilities like the RN, but they also perform specific medical assignments. Also, an LPN has to work under the supervision of an RN. An LPN program takes almost a year to complete. An LPN examines patients, observe critical symptoms, and assist in wound care. Examples of facilities where LPNs work are hospitals, home health care, nursing homes, and clinics.

The Registered nurses (RN) have, at least, a two-year degree or three-year diploma. Most of them have baccalaureate degrees. RNs also have a wide range of experience and advanced skills due to their training. They are more frequently employed in hospital settings compared to the LPNs. Registered Nurses are mostly expected to engage in critical thinking while performing their tasks.

As a Registered nurse, you have to perform multiple tasks, most of which includes attending to all the needs of your patients, ensuring that they get adequate comfort in a safe and secure environment. As an RN, you are expected to observe and take note of instructions given by the doctors and accomplish each task appropriately. RNs are tasked with the responsibility of carrying out advanced medical modalities and functions such as assessing their patients to know all the relevant information, thereby developing care plans applicable to their health status. It's no wonder why RNs are majorly the key search when employers are seeking nurses to hire. Besides providing immediate care when required, RNs also take leadership roles and apply critical thinking to deliver appropriate medical services.

- **How do LPNs and RNs attain their educational status, and what tasks/ jobs can they do?**

To answer this question comprehensively, it is better to highlight the variety of aspects as related to their education, curriculum, workplace, the scope of practice, their roles and responsibilities, and potential earning.

1) **LPN and RN According to the Education** - The process of becoming an LPN and RN is different. What determines the certificate you attain is the path you choose at the beginning of your studies. As an RN student, it takes two to three years to complete the program, by which you will be awarded a Bachelor of Nursing (BSN). As for an aspiring LPN student, he or she is required to finish the program in one year. LPN Students are either awarded a diploma or certificate in nursing, depending on the institution.

Most people are indecisive about what they intend to do when considering their career prospects. This is why it is recommended to consult an education counselor to know which path is suitable for you. Although the decision is entirely up to you, you need an experienced person to guide you as you make your choice. The better the clarity you have for you, the rewarding it will be for you. The goal is to get a job with security and satisfaction. Just be specific about what you want when setting your career goals.

The requirement for an LPN program is a high school diploma or GED, after which you will have to complete nine to eighteen (9 – 18) months of the program. On completing this stage, you are mean to pass a state licensing assessment paper. The education equips you to assist a Registered Nurse in a medical unit.

A requirement for aspiring RN students is a bachelor or associate degree from an accredited nursing school. The education equips you to function in the management department of the health sector. Further studies can also reward you a leadership position. Most education counselors will recommend you follow his path.

2) **LPN and RN According to the Scope of Practice** - For a licensed practical nurse, the scope of practice is limited. This is not the same for the registered nurse, who is permitted to manage the entire nursing staff and function independently without having to report to other nurses. It takes a very long process for an LPN to attain this level of responsibility. Additional scope of practice includes:

Licensed practical nurse work under the supervision of registered nurses and other physicians. LPNs also have the opportunity to become registered nurses after a few working experiences. However, it can be a bit tough trying to continue education after a period of medical practice. It takes strong determination and commitment to achieve that.

Registered Nurses have a lot of career prospect, especially after obtaining a master degree (MSN). Positions like nurse administrator, nurse practitioner, nurse educator, and specialist nurse are available to a registered nurse. There is a lot of opportunism for the RNs as they advance their studies. For instance, obtaining a doctorate degree opens the RNs to opportunities in administration, careers in practice, policy, and education.

Registered nurses also participate in specialized practices. Registered nurses have more career opportunities compared to licensed practical nurses.

3) **LPN and RN According to their Workplace** - A lot of licensed practical nurses work in long term care, more than in any other setting. In time, they will have opportunities to advance in the nursing hierarchy – from supervising nursing assistant who perform most rudimentary duties. In 2011, the NLN reported that newly licensed Practical nurses in long term care were almost 6 times as likely to function in an administrative capacity as the registered nurses.

In health care facilities, you will find that licensed practical nurses have limited advancement opportunities. They also do not have many options for specialization.

According to the Bureau of Labor Statistics (BLS) reports, 48% are in private facilities, 29 percent of licensed practical nurses work in nursing care facilities, 15% in hospitals, others in doctor's office, local hospitals and home health centers.

When you discover that a particular hospital is more beneficial to target for employment, you should go for it.

4) **LPN and RN According to their Duties** - Duties of registered nurses: RNs perform more advanced tasks because of their advanced training. These duties are planning of care, patient's education, administering medications, critical thinking, patients' assessments, handoff documentation, etc. Registered nurses also take orders from doctors and make a treatment plan. Registered nurses are responsible for the LPNs, that is, they schedule the work of the licensed practical nurses.

The roles and responsibilities of an RN are further listed below:

- Registered nurses are responsible for coordinating the medical staff, including assigning duties to a certified nurse assistants (CNA) and LPN and among others.

- Apart from prescribing medications and giving treatment, registered nurses inform the patients and their family members about relevant details that will improve their health conditions. They also provide emotional support to their patients.

- Due to their advanced training, registered nurses know a lot about all the equipment and the best ways on how to use them.

- Based on the assessment of patients and consultations with the physicians, the registered nurse administers treatment to patients. These assessments are done by checking temperature, blood pressure, and taking diagnostic tests to ascertain the extent of the health condition. RNs carry out these tests and analyze the outcomes.

- Registered nurses are responsible for preparing the plan for the treatment of patients.

- While registered nurses are responsible for complex tasks and more advanced way of caring for the patients, the licensed practical nurses are restricted to the basics. LPNs only perform a complex if they are guided by a more experienced medical staff.

Duties of the LPNs - The roles of the licensed practical nurses are limited compared to the RNs. They carry out tasks such as taking blood pressure, carrying out orders from registered nurses, they monitor the health status of patients, treat injuries, changes bandage and inserts flexible tube leading to the bladder through the narrow opening, assist patients in bathing and getting dressed up and so many others.

LPNs are also responsible for patient education to some extent. They do this by discussing their health conditions with them and highlight possible improvement strategies. They listen to the patient to know what they have to say, they reach out to their patients psychologically, etc.

Licensed practical nurses also take orders and report back to registered nurses and doctors.

LPN nurses keep track of the progress or health status of the patients when it is required.

An experienced licensed practical nurse can direct and manage new graduate LPNs and medical staffs with minimal or no clinical experience or license.

IMPORTANT QUESTIONS YOU SHOULD ASK YOURSELF BEFORE DECIDING TO BECOME A NURSE

If you are interested in practicing nursing full time, then it is also highly essential that you understand what your daily responsibilities will be and whether or not you'll be able to cope with the responsibilities.

As an aspiring nurse, understand that the nursing profession varies according to the scope of practice.

For example, the scope of practice as a nurse attorney or nurse entrepreneur is different from those of an ER nurse or nurse practitioner. When giving your feedback to the listed questions, identify whether or not they apply to your chosen career field.

Majority of these questions will focus on general nursing, but may also apply to other areas of nursing.

MENTAL

As a nurse, you will deal with several psychological stresses in your work routine.

Here is a list of questions you should ask yourself to help you determine whether or not you will be comfortable dealing with the stresses as related.

✓ **Do you enjoy interacting with people on a daily basis?**

As a licensed nurse, you will need to have excellent interpersonal skills and be able to communicate regularly with your patients and coworkers daily.

Your ability to communicate with other members of your unit will be tested at the initial stage of your work.

Communicating effectively with your patients and colleagues will be extremely important in the nursing practice.

✓ **Do you work well with a team?**

The nursing practice is team-oriented. The complex nature of the job requires multiple heads and hands at stake. Assistant nurses, LPNs, RNs, and other physicians work together to ensure the safety of patients.

The ability to work efficiently and function well as a member of a team is vital.

Working with a team transcends just communicating with them.

You have responsibilities such as coordinating tasks, taking the lead on projects, assist the LPNs in implementing the tasks, etc.

✓ **Are you passionate about helping people improve their mental and physical health status?**

A registered nurse is responsible for duties such as patients' education, administering treatments and medications to patients. Some of the things you're going to teach them include, how to improve their medical condition, side effects of some drugs, how to take dosages of specific drugs and other essential facts for their care and safety.

As a nurse, you are also responsible for documenting medical information on patients, addressing patients' concerns, assessing patients' health status, performing medical procedures, and so on.

✓ **Do you have good organizational skills?**

Keeping track of your tasks in a very orderly manner is one of your duties as a nurse.

Organize your tasks in order of priorities to enable you to complete them effectively and in time. You patients' medical records should also be appropriately documented.

Medical equipment should be well organized after use. You can direct your LPNs to carry out such tasks. Enter information in patients' chart legibly and orderly.

Disorganized work will contribute to your stress and make you prone to critical errors. Having good organizational skill will prevent any complication.

✓ **Can you work well under stressful situations?**

Some days can be so full of activities that you will keep standing on your feet several hours at a stretch.

For instance, nurses that work in the ER or critical care unit may have to care for several patients that are suffering from life-threatening illnesses, psychological disorders, or physical injuries.

The ability to manage your patients efficiently without getting distracted or feeling overwhelmed mentally is vital towards the patients' safety.

✓ **Can you manage your time effectively?**

Time management is a very essential factor in nursing practice.

Punctuality, prioritizing your tasks, conducting your handoffs promptly and in order, performing medical tasks carefully and effectively, etc. are all responsibilities that come with the job.

Managing time efficiently give you an avenue to finish your task and have time to rest. Encroaching into the time allotted for an on-coming patient can cause conflict, you may have to avoid that.

✓ **Do you have good listening skills?**

During work hours, the environment gets so busy that it becomes difficult to concentrate. It takes an experienced nurse to deal with such stress excellently well.

Busy hours are often filled with commotions, but if you can maintain your calm and attend to your tasks without losing attention, mistakes will be avoided.

Being a good listener is a quality that can be learned. It is not a gift. Your patient may not want to shout, the doctor may be having a migraine headache, under these circumstances, try to listen attentively.

Excellent listening skills are an essential asset in medical practice.

✓ **Can you juggle multiple tasks effectively?**

Nurses handle multiple complex situations regularly. It's a common challenge that comes with the job.

Under this situation, you need to cut off all forms of distractions – phones have to be switched off, interactions with colleagues have to be tuned down to allow you focus. Losing concentration can lead to a fatal mistake.

You also need to turn off media devices if it's in the room where you are carrying out your tasks. Managing different patients at this same time requires all the concentration you need.

✓ **Are you comfortable with reading, researching, and writing for long periods of time?**

Activities such as research, record keeping, and reading information to physicians during patients' education are aspects of medical practice required to make medical care efficient.

To be able to engage in side jobs like blogging or content writing for nursing publications requires research and dedication to studies.

EMOTIONAL

One of the most neglected aspects of nursing profession is comprehending the emotional responsibilities nurses experience on a daily basis.

As you continually attend to your patients, you get attached to them emotionally. Most time, you can't help it. Nurses are compassionate by nature. To be able to connect with patients and develop an emotional connection is often natural. This is why the loss of a patient can deal a significant blow to nurses who were very close to the deceased.

Another source of concern is raising conflicts between coworkers. Conflicts are inevitable no matter how contained you think they are. It can affect performance because the mind is not in its best.

Here are some questions to ask yourself when it comes to dealing with the emotional components of nursing practice:

✓ **Are you able to take the lead when other team members are absent or less experienced?**

Registered nurses are taught leadership skills in nursing schools. You should be able to translate what you've learned practically in the organization.

✓ **When you are faced with circumstances where you'll have to take the lead on executing specific tasks or are responsible for educating new nurses about their responsibilities and how to perform effectively will you be comfortable with leading?**

✓ **How well do you manage interpersonal conflicts?**

Your priority as a nurse is with the care and wellbeing of the patients.

When there's a rising conflict, your professional values are called to question. You should be able to keep your emotional outbursts in check.

Don't be quick to react. Understand that opinions always vary. Don't expect too much of people. Your reactions and ability to keep things under control defines who you are. Being able to put your differences aside and work together to accomplish your tasks at hand will be incredibly invaluable in the workplace.

When you notice that the issue is way over your head, how you react is very vital.

✓ **Will you talk to human resources or your manager to try and resolve the conflict, will you lash out at your coworker or find another way to handle the situation?**

You will need to be able to find another way.

✓ **Does the thought of dealing with bodily fluids such as blood, vomit, urine, or feces bother you?**

If the thought of handling blood, urine, vomit, feces, or other bodily fluids irritates you, you should seriously reconsider the right nursing field for you. Although you can work anywhere as a nurse after you are licensed during clinicals you will be expected to provide bodily care.

✓ **How do you emotionally deal with severely injured or sick patients?**

Working in an environment where there are severely injured patient(s) shouldn't pose a problem for a real nurse. The only reaction that should come from you is that of sympathy and compassion.

If your emotions will get in the way of your performance, seek help from an expert. Nurses feel satisfied when they notice that a patient they have been working with recovers from an illness or injury. Experience can play a vital role in dealing with complex or rare medical cases

✓ **Are you able to work effectively despite getting connected emotionally to some of your patients?**

As a nurse, it is difficult for nurses to not get emotionally attached to their patients. Caring for a patient for a long time makes you susceptible to emotional attachments.

The relationship takes another phase when the patients go into recovery. It could end at the door or continue depending on the kind of person involved. However, emotional attachments should have positive outcome rather than negative. When you bond well with your patients, you feel excited about going to your job, or in their rooms. Emotional attachment is also a form of trust.

✓ **Do you have a lot of patience?**

Nurses possess the virtue of patience. Either you're working as a forensic nurse talking to victims and witnesses, gathering information or working as a registered nurse talking to your patients to understand their condition you may find yourself spending lots of time on specific tasks that require a lot of patience and understanding.

If you work in a nursing home or rehabilitation center, for instance, you will have to adjust to a slower pace of care, than you may be used to.

In the medical practice, listening and patience are two crucial components to providing quality patient care.

✓ **Are you into practice for the money or because you're passionate about nursing and healthcare?**

A standard answer to interview question of this nature, gets answers like this, "no sir, my major driving force is the passion I have for the job." This may seem like a wise answer, but it lacks originality. Be sincere about your answers.

Also, if your primary or only motivation is financial benefits, then you may quickly lose interest in the nursing profession.

A certain level of passion is the anchor that keeps people committed to a job even when money is no forthcoming.

Your primary reason for becoming a nurse should be as a result of emotional interest instead of financial benefits.

PHYSICAL

The nursing profession also requires physical input. Health care services are not sent via Bluetooth or downloaded online without human involvement.

The following lists of questions to give you better clarity on what you'll have to deal with physically as a nurse.

✓ **Are you okay with working long hours and/or working morning, noon, and night shifts?**

Some private healthcare facilities have policies that make it mandatory for nurses to work long hours at a stretch.

If you ever find yourself in a growing organization where staffs are insufficient, it's possible to be asked that kind of question.

In addition to this, some fields of nursing require staffing 24 hours a day, and you may be required to work morning, noon, and/or night shifts.

Such a question can also be meant to test your commitment capacity.

✓ **If you work for a department or healthcare center that requires this sort of flexibility, are you comfortable working these types of hours?**

Can you cope with the physical demands of standing on your feet for long hours? During busy periods, nurses spend long hours walking on their feet.

Physical activities such as handling medical equipment, answering phone calls, coordinating with other team members and moving between the work station and the patient area, etc. could keep you on your feet at a long stretch.

✓ **Are you ok with physically moving people regularly?**

It is common in a large health care facility for nurses and family members to move a patient from place to place inside the hospital environment. Moving patients is a common task within some areas of nursing.

✓ **Are you able to move heavy equipment on a regular basis?**

It's also possible to carry heavy hospital equipment from place to place. You have to understand how your body responds to physical stress to avoid causing a breakdown.

Equipment with wheels may be easy to move, but, others may require more energy to push or lift.

Lifting heavy loads can affect the joints or pelvic region.

All of these questions will help you discover if nursing is right for you!

Final Thoughts

I started my nursing career as a teenager taking care of my two very sick grandparents.

They required an in-home skilled nurse practitioner to perform tasks such as bed baths, blood sugar checks, and wound dressing changes.

The nurse just happened to be a 16-year old girl.

It was through a caring home health nurse named Linda that I learned the physical acts make nurses so important to healthcare. Having a mentor for this type of education made my growth in knowledge exciting and manageable. She taught me how to care for the people I loved in a competent and effective way.

I didn't have Linda when I started my first nursing professional job so my transition was not so smooth. But what I learned then has now allowed me to have an exceptional and amazing nursing career.

I hope that all I have shared will encourage and motivate you to take your nursing career to the highest level possible.

You are needed, you are the future of nursing, the world is waiting to embrace what you have to offer!

Sincerely,

Regina Callion MSN, RN

Founder, CEO - ReMarNurse.com